Ian Rogers
Frederick L. Vanderbom

The Consequence And Cause Of Pyloric Stenosis Of Infancy

Ian Rogers
Frederick L. Vanderbom

The Consequence And Cause Of Pyloric Stenosis Of Infancy

Two Personal Stories

LAP LAMBERT Academic Publishing

Imprint

Any brand names and product names mentioned in this book are subject to trademark, brand or patent protection and are trademarks or registered trademarks of their respective holders. The use of brand names, product names, common names, trade names, product descriptions etc. even without a particular marking in this work is in no way to be construed to mean that such names may be regarded as unrestricted in respect of trademark and brand protection legislation and could thus be used by anyone.

Cover image: www.ingimage.com

Publisher:
LAP LAMBERT Academic Publishing
is a trademark of
International Book Market Service Ltd., member of OmniScriptum Publishing Group
17 Meldrum Street, Beau Bassin 71504, Mauritius

ISBN: 978-3-659-52125-6

Copyright © Ian Rogers, Frederick L. Vanderbom
Copyright © 2014 International Book Market Service Ltd., member of OmniScriptum Publishing Group

The Consequence and Cause of Pyloric Stenosis of Infancy

Two Personal Stories

Table of Contents

The Consequence

My Personal Story—Rev. Fred. L. Vanderbom B.A.(Hons)

                                                                Pages 4-22.

The Cause

My Personal Story—Ian Rogers F.R.C.S., F.R.C.P.

Personal History - gastrin and acid.   Pages 23-30

The Cause of Infantile Hypertrophic Pyloric Stenosis.(I.H.P.S.)

The clinical clues	**Pages 30-31**
The Historical setting.	**Pages 32-33**

My Journey.

Neonatal gastrin and acid.	Pages 33-37
Pyloric sphincter contraction.	Pages 37
Physiology of gastric emptying in the adult.	Pages 37-40
Gastric function and the hyperacidity theory.	Pages 40-42.
I.H.P.S. and Acid Secretion.	Pages 42-44
Sphincter work hypertrophy as the cause.	Pages 44-46
The Anatomy/Pathology of Sphincter Hypertrophy	Pages 46-47
The Motilin Story.	Pages 47-48

Clinical Aspects. — **Pages 48-49**

Clinical Questions Resolved. — **Pages 49**

Q.1. Why do babies develop IHPS?	Pages 50-52
Supporting evidence for hyperacidity.	Pages 52
Q.2. Why male babies?	Pages 53
Q.3. Why self-cure with time?	Pages 54-58
Q.4. Why more frequent in the first born?	Pages 58
Q.5. Why does the tumour disappear after pyloro-myotomy and not after gastro-enterostomy?	Pages 59
Q.6. Why do symptoms appear at 3-4 weeks?	Pages 59-60

Other Contemporary Lines of Enquiry.	**Pages 60**
The Genetic Story	Pages 60-61
Growth Factors and Chemical Agents.	Pages 61
The Infection Theories.	Pages 61-62
Conclusion.	**Pages 63**
The Future.	**Pages 63-64**
References,Acknowledgements/Biodata.	**Pages 64-71**

The Consequence

My Story – Fred Vanderbom

I would have been known as "Fountain Fred" within ten days after I was born. I had pyloric stenosis almost from birth: not just the "wet burps" and some reflux that all babies have.

The opening piece of this tome is my personal account of infant hypertrophic pyloric stenosis, the weird condition that causes between two and five tiny babies in every 1,000 to vomit violently and uncontrollably, how this condition and infant surgery have affected me and some others, and how pyloric stenosis in babies can be recognized more promptly and treated better than it so often is.

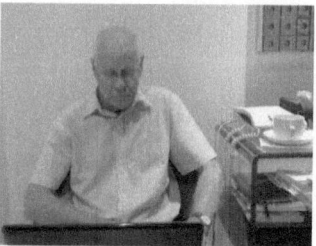

What I have written here has been edited from a "page" of my blog, *Surviving Infant Surgery*[1]. I started blogging about infant hypertrophic pyloric stenosis ("PS") early in 2011 as a retirement project to grow understanding and air my own and others' personal stories among patients and parents who have been or are being touched by pyloric stenosis. During three years the number of reader "visits" to my blog has risen to almost 70 per day and totals 50,000 over that period.

I have found that reading and writing for this blog is not only therapeutic; it is also adding in a small way to the wider awareness of the issues around this horrible, all-too-common but hardly known and all-too-often poorly diagnosed condition. Its consequences for a minority of those affected is scantily understood and managed. Some of the Comments on my blogsite and elsewhere on web forums are very heart-rending.

Here I want to give a brief overview of what pyloric stenosis looks like and how it's treated, very much in the light of something of my story. Click on an image if it's too small for you to get its message. Many of these images are taken from the web and have been used in my posts.

This is what pyloric stenosis looks like . . .

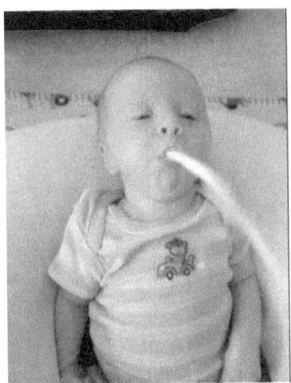

Ewww... yuck, Fred!

Yeah, but in 1945, even grainy black-and-white photos were hardly affordable to my War-weary parents... so this web image will have to remind us that pyloric stenosis is a truly scary condition that can end a baby's short life within weeks if not days. I was born in a small "city" (with just a few thousand inhabitants but city status) in the northern Dutch province of Friesland. As happened there and then, being a church minister my proud father paid somebody to announce my birth to all the town notables... my parents clearly felt pleased, honoured, relieved and grateful to God. They even kept the receipt for this service (7.50 Dutch florins) …

Translation: *Received from the honourable Mr Reverend Bom [sic] the sum of 7.50 florins for the public announcement of the birth of their son. A Hagersma*

Despite this anecdote it is hard to imagine how devastated my parents must have felt when the violent vomiting that is pyloric stenosis started a few days later. I have read that some tiny pyloric stenosis bubs can shoot milk one or two metres (yards) and perhaps further. Soon it was clear that I was vomiting myself to exhaustion and death when only a week old. The violence of a stenotic pylorus puking can cause bleeding in the stomach, give rise to herniation of the abdominal wall and even damage the brain.

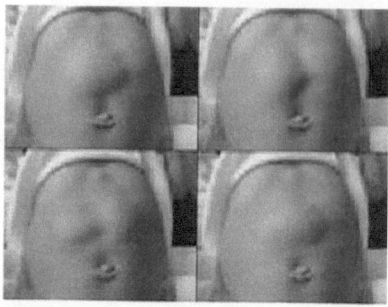

This is not me either but I would have caused both interest and consternation when my belly performed like this... A clear sign of pyloric stenosis is that you can see the stomach muscles trying to push food (waves of peristalsis) through the overgrown and blocked pyloric valve at the end of the stomach.

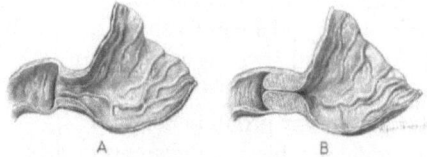

"Pylorus" is Greek for "gate", and in pyloric stenosis, the normal stomach's exit gate muscle (A) becomes thickened (B), narrowing ('stenosing") and then often blocking the stomach's exit passage. The cause is too much acid in the passage over-stimulating the muscle, but all this is still only very partially understood.

Maternal stress, several genes, milk chemistry, an antibiotic, and over-feeding or formula feeding are among the suspects. In 2012 and 2013 reports from Denmark[2] and the United States[3] on thorough studies implicated bottle feeding as a risk factor, and its chemistry is different from breast milk. Some earlier reports have claimed that bottle feeding reduces the risk of pyloric stenosis, perhaps because it made quantity easier to control. Some statistics say older mothers are at greater risk of having a pyloric stenosis baby, more recent studies claim to have found a youthful first birth is more at risk, and yet others say maternal age is not a factor. Some reports have prematurity as a risk factor and others not. In other words, some risk factors are clear and others are still debated after several hundred years of PS being recognized.

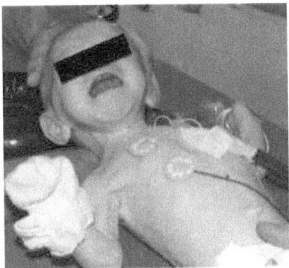

Again, not me! How I would like there to have been photos and journal jottings of what happened to me back in 1945 – but they were very different times.

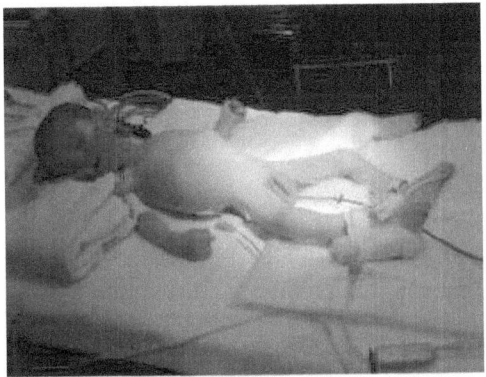

This and the previous distressing web images show the dangerous hunger and dehydration which pyloric stenosis all-too-often causes before it is diagnosed and managed.

Many parents report how very angry and frustrated they were when their doctors stalled deciding on what had become obvious to them, especially if they themselves had had pyloric stenosis or if the condition had surfaced earlier in their family, or after they'd done their own careful homework.

But parents also need to realize that pyloric stenosis can sometimes be hard to distinguish from other gastric complaints. Many regret that the more recently trained doctors no longer follow the traditional clinical steps to reach an initial diagnosis: there are several clear physical signs of pyloric stenosis and perhaps a family history which together usually give a strong indication of this condition, and x-ray and ultrasound examinations were only used in the past when the clinical diagnosis was uncertain. Now, judging by countless reports, too many GPs and paediatricians belittle parents, talk about "alternative diagnoses" and wait until the costly technologies can be considered justified, all in the name of "the scientific approach" – although one may wonder whether the training, politics, fears and cashflow of the medical industry also play a part.

Is it any wonder there are so many stories on the web of parents despairing of their doctor and taking their expiring baby to the local hospital's Emergency Department – only to be told: "If you had brought your baby in any later, (s)he wouldn't have made the night"?

Many pyloric stenosis babies don't get to this distressing state before they are diagnosed. But many mothers well know when their baby is actually losing ground, that this is serious, and that they are not being treated with due respect. Their stories are too numerous to be brushed aside.

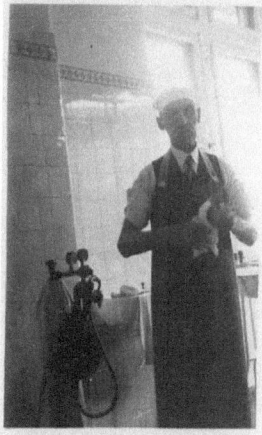

This workmanlike guy deserves pride of place here: the German Dr Conrad Ramstedt doesn't look like an eminent surgeon when judged by today's dress codes, but in back in 1911 he discovered and in 1912 (over a century ago now, yay!) he published the simple remedy for projectile vomiting. And ... he'd discovered it partly by accident, partly through good observation and thinking.[4]

I owe my life to Dr Conrad Ramstedt.

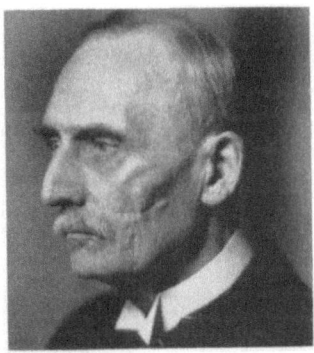

Another and more distinguished looking photo of Dr Ramstedt. He started his medical career in the German Army. It looks like he suffered some collateral damage – mebbee in a sword fight in Cavalry training? "Can I stick to medicine now, Colonel?"

RAMSTEDT'S OPERATION

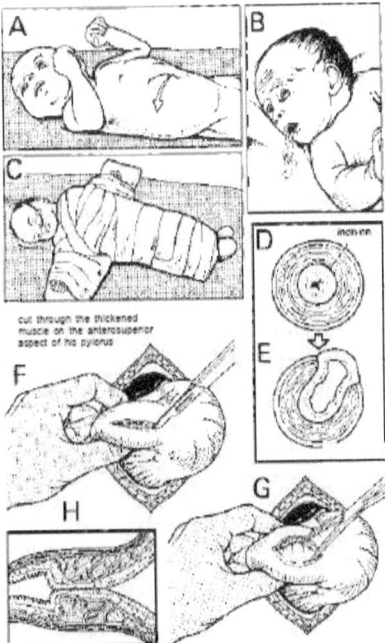

This 1950s series shows how the Ramstedt pyloromyotomy for pyloric stenosis was (and often still is) done, by open surgery.

What this set doesn't tell us is that anesthesia for babies was primitive and dangerous until the 1960s, and often avoided until the late 1980s, something that has had lasting effects on some of us who have struggled lifelong with various degrees of Post Traumatic Stress Disorder ("PTSD").

In my case in the Netherlands in 1945, it was commonplace to be given some local anesthetic injected around the incision site and perhaps a sugar cube (sometimes supercharged with brandy) to keep the baby quiet (or try to?). Until recent decades, most babies having surgery were not given a general anesthetic but were intubated (they had a breathing tube pushed down their throat) and were then given a paralysing drug to keep them from writhing with the surgery. Of course my mind doesn't remember any of this... but it is becoming increasingly recognized that babies do feel pain and that although the newborn brain is too little developed to remember trauma, the body can be affected in a lasting way.[5]

Pyloromyotomy (splitting the pyloric muscle) has become *the* favourite operation of many surgeons: it is simple, quick, and usually immediately and obviously effective. Traumatised and anxious parents may hug the infant's surgical team for a miracle change.

But older surgeons had to be trained to disregard the clear signs of great distress during infant surgery, as only a very few surgeons with teams in large hospitals had the skills to give a baby a safe general anesthetic. "At least we're saving this baby's life... the parents will be grateful, and so one day should this child!"

Specialist pediatric anesthesia was only born in 1949[6] and developed very slowly, so it was convenient that it was generally believed that babies don't remember pain and are not affected by it. However, the 1987 study by Dr K J S Anand showed conclusively that this is not so[7]. It has only been over the past 25 years that the standard practice has become that under 2 year olds are given a general anesthetic for any surgical procedure. Circumcision remains a late stronghold of old shibboleths.

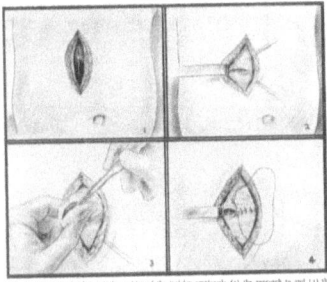

My op was done just like these drawings show, except that I was cut down my middle rather than just to the right of centre (upper para-midline) as in these drawings. This drawing prompted me to discover the buried scar from the transverse incision under my vertical scar (illustrations 2 & 4). A dehiscence (wound rupture) is more likely with vertical midline abdominal incisions and is to be avoided. Dehiscence was once a fairly common complication.

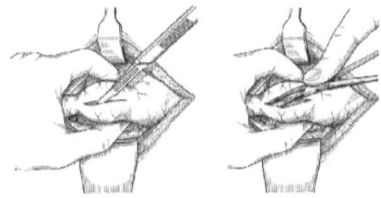

Another internet drawing of what happens in a pyloromyotomy. The thickened muscle band around the stomach outlet (left pic) has become 1-2 cm long, whitish, and very hard (sometimes like cartilage), blocking everything. It is slit and then prised to gape open length-wise down to the mucosa, the inner lining of the passage. Keeping the mucosa intact and not damaging the duodenum are vital: any leak has to be identified and repaired before the wound's closure. There are several videos showing a pyloromyotomy on YouTube.
And yay! My stressed-out Mother's milk could get through. "Ramstedt's operation" is known as "most elegant surgery": a quick, simple, almost bloodless, and usually effective fix with nothing removed or rearranged.

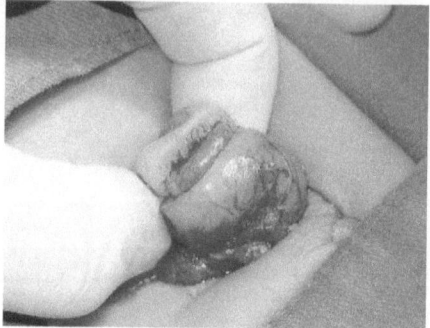

Another photo from the web – this little gash through the overgrown muscle is what saves most pyloric stenosis babies today from a slow death by dehydration and starvation. This is the gist of the pyloric stenosis repair – the enlarged pylorus muscle has been split to open wide, but the lining of the gastric passage is left intact. Bring on the food! Like many pyloric stenosis babies I flourished after my op... just look at the 3rd pikkie below here.

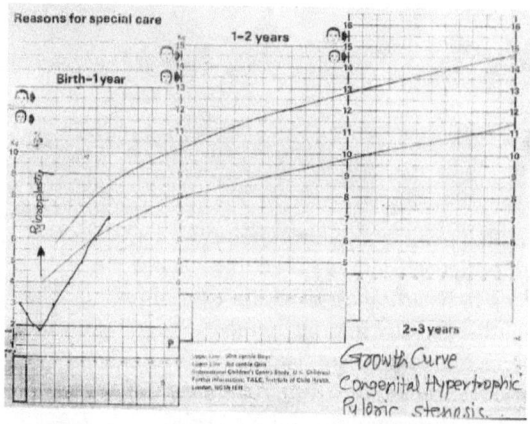

My parents dumped all the records of my pyloric stenosis story (grrrr), but I remember them having a weight chart which looked very much like this one, with a steep dip bottoming at 10 days (not 2 months) – followed by a rapid rise. Whooppee – my pylorus learnt the severe lesson: it seems it was so keen to avoid further punishment that it obligingly let my intake pass through very quickly – which enhanced my ability to eat as much as I liked without a weight problem.

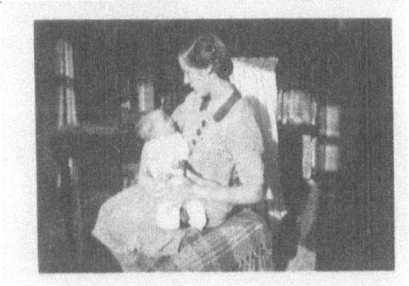

A bit more about me. This is most likely the first photo of me – being held by a clearly concerned Mum. And yes, it's very basic.

I was born just four months after the Second World War ended, and after an even longer dark time for my parents. Mum and Dad had endured a 7 year engagement due first to the Depression and then the German occupation of their country. Then, 10 days after my arrival they had to hand their firstborn over for what was by today's standards rough and ready surgery to remedy my uncontrollable vomiting – followed by several weeks of maternal separation in hospital because of the danger of infection (2-3 weeks was the norm). Every day Ma had to travel 15 km to the hospital by steam train to deliver some breast milk. Must have been fun times for my parents. Is it any wonder they decided never to talk about all this?

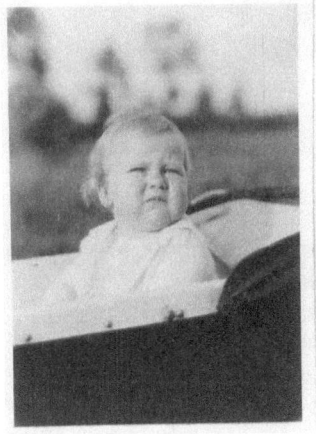

But here's the good news: I survived and flourished. Half a year after my operation (and probably already at half a month) I was looking very healthy, thank you. Many pyloric stenosis babies quickly make up their weight loss and go to the top of their percentile range.

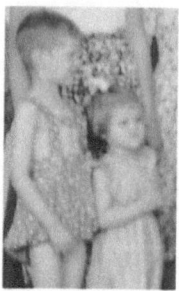

It's now April 1951 – and this fuzzy photo shows not a sign yet of the trauma and manic phobia I developed during the next year, when I came to fear anyone seeing and asking me about the gnarled scar down my middle. Mum made her four kids these cute summer suits in several sizes; they were of a standard design in those austere post-War times (and I've seen several of them on photos from that era) – with a neat window for the top half of my belly scar to peek through.

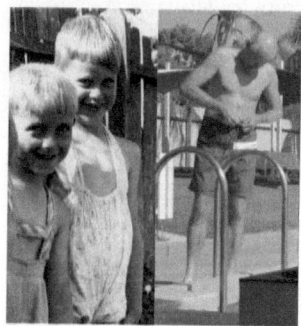

Not only women have self-image issues: some of us guys also take years to stop hating our body. My temperament didn't help; I'm such an earnest and perfectionist builder/ retriever/ beaver. By age 6 years (as is common) I had become self-conscious and obsessed about the stomach scar I got as a baby. Mum then made me a special new summer outfit with a waist rather higher and unhip than her earlier design which has now been handed down to my brother. I look very pleased with the new gear, but it only delayed the issues I would have to deal with.

I wish now that my parents had done more to help me to understand and "own" my life-saving story. There is so much reason to be thankful to God, my doctor and my parents that I
- was born in a time and place that allowed me to survive a stomach blockage,
- have been able to come to terms with many of the symptoms of mild PTSD,
- am reminded daily of the fact that all of us humans struggle with our brokenness,
- now feel proud of being marked with what represents a lifesaver, and
- belong to a worldwide community of people with a pyloric stenosis story to tell.

During my school years I showed what I now recognise as the signs of PTSD, although they were mild and without suicidal tendencies. In the 1950s the word "trauma" was hardly heard: soldiers suffered from "shell shock" and it seemed so many women had depression problems, but everybody was told that "time heals everything", "you'd better get over it", and "just get on with your life".

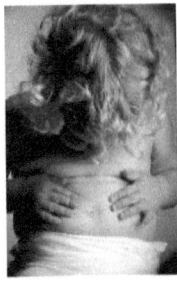

Sadly, it doesn't usually work that way. I grew up in a secret world of –
- self-obsession (I'm sure I wore out a few mirrors and certainly wasted loads of time),
- self-injuring (I learnt a lot and am thankful I did myself no lasting harm), and
- searching libraries for anything to explain my scar and what caused it.
- I discovered that I was fearful of especially doctors but also of anyone I regarded as in authority, and became passive-aggressive, internalising my anger.
- Although I have functioned quite well in my work and relationships I am also known as the sole reserved, introverted reclusive in my immediate family of seven and even my extended family.

- I love the water but at the pool and beach I never felt able to relax and enjoy myself except actually in the water. For many years when out of the water I would keep my arms tightly folded to hide my scar from curious eyes and tug my shorts or swimmers up to my chest, forever annoying my mother who kept reminding me that this looked ridiculous – which I didn't really care about as much as...
- I lied, denied and pleaded ignorance when people did ask me what "that" was on my belly or what my scar was from. I avoided phys-ed classes at school, sports and overnight camps which involved changing or showering in public, and my face blushed and heart raced whenever I heard any of a short but telling list of words.

During my late teens and courtship it took me several years (yes!) to summon the courage to tell my best friend and life partner about my pyloric stenosis and scar – only to find that they were no big deal to her; besides this she told me of a niece who had had the same condition and operation.

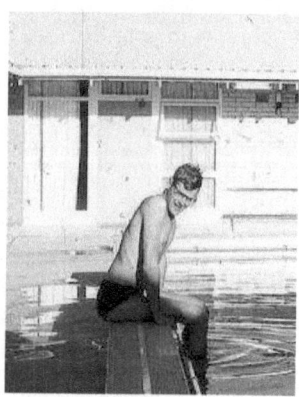

Yet even during our honeymoon this poolside pose shows how careful I was about showing my belly to the world. It has taken me many years to feel as free, proud and grateful to God and my family and friends as I do now because I survived something that used to take the life of most babies who had it.

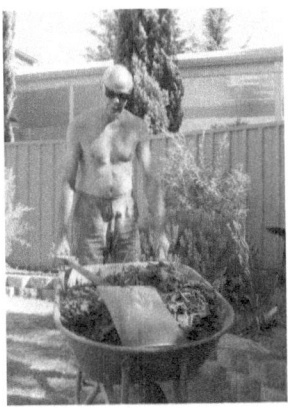

Despite always being a beanpole and now watching my weight, I've added a bit of flab in recent years and my scar has become even more indented, a common look. It's become clearer that adhesions have also glued it to my insides. I've learnt much about my pyloric stenosis story and how I've reacted to it – but regrettably, the details and my parents' vital part in it will remain a blank almost totally. Their lips remained sealed, sadly to their graves and the medical records were shredded many years ago.

I do hope that every parent of a "PSer" will be able to do much more today to help their child to know, understand and embrace their story.

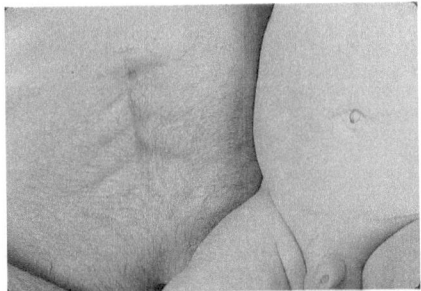

This photo from a German medical website[8] is very special to me. The father on the left has almost a clone of my scar, and his son had a fairly recent laparoscopic pyloric stenosis operation. This image was posted to show the progress pyloric stenosis surgery has made since 1980 when a baby's belly was still routinely and often roughly slit open and then sewn up like a football with big black threads.

Networking with others sharing my story has assured me that although still generally dismissed as "impossible", it's far from abnormal to be left with some emotional baggage from surgery which we cannot remember but which has affected us in ways that parents would rather not know about or forget and which doctors tend to brush off or ignore.

Several pyloromyotomy scars I have seen, including the one above and my own (below) have a hollow somewhere along the incision line, quite visible if you click on this 1968 slide photo. I wonder if (despite several denials online to other curious survivors) a drain was sometimes left in the wound?

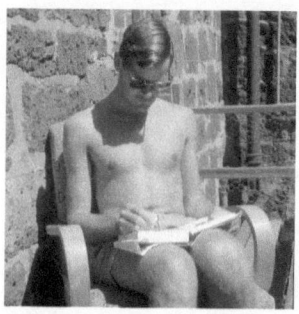

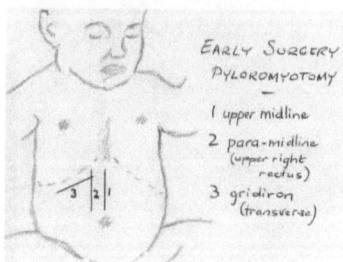

Prof Dr Conrad Ramstedt liked the upper midline incision for the best access to his pyloromyotomy, whilst other surgeons came to favour other incisions as they result in fewer complications: the upper para-midline, the Kocher (subcostal, or angled under the right ribs), and transverse (horizontal) incisions in the upper right quadrant. Whatever the choice, for many years an old-style magnified Kanji-like scar from this operation was the give-away sign for old-school doctors that their patient had probably survived pyloric stenosis.

During the past 15 years, it has become easier (and some might say fashionable) to respect cosmetic considerations: the surgical repair of pyloric stenosis is now often been done via between one and four 2-4 mm laparoscopic probes, or via a small incision around or through the umbilicus. Surgeons who still work through an open incision usually prefer a transverse incision (although all the old favourites still seem to be in occasional use), and the stitches that close the wound are almost always subcutaneous (buried under the skin at the edges of the incision): this leaves a much tidier scar, as this beautifully captured image from the *Life Lines* blog[9] shows.

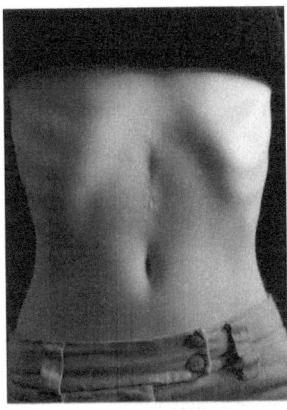

However, although laparoscopic pyloric stenosis surgery doesn't leave much damage at first, by school age the probes' scars can become several navel-like pits on the abdomen: as someone has commented, "My belly looks as if it's taken a shrapnel hit".

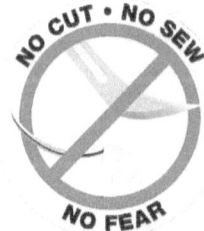

Reports from several developed but non-English speaking countries show that between 70 and 85% of pyloric stenosis babies will actually respond to medical (anti-acid) treatment with the drug atropine or now Ranitidine which relaxes the pyloric muscle until the baby's growth takes its own care of pyloric stenosis. Although medical drug treatment is not without hazards and takes a little coaching of the parents and a course of several weeks, it has been used worldwide for over a century and is safe and non-traumatic for both the parents and the baby... and the surgery option can always be taken up if necessary.

The vast majority of infant PS patients recover quickly from their surgery with no, minimal or manageable side-effects. The same is true of the ongoing physical and emotional effects of PS and pyloromyotomy on adult life. However, from my personal experience and 17 years of following this subject closely using the medical and personal resources available via the internet, it has become very clear that there is a substantial number of people who do have significant ongoing difficulties which are (often quite clearly) attributable to their surgery. From the mass of material which can be traced or read online these sequelae have been researched not at all or only very scantily, and are thus disregarded by most physicians.

One of my blog's "messages" is that conservative or medical treatment should be the first option for most pyloric stenosis babies older than 3 weeks.

Do I have other dreams on my wish-list? Almost thought you'd never ask... here are some –
- More frequent good diagnosis of infant pyloric stenosis, supported by a better understanding of what makes for good patient – doctor relations.
- Growing clarity and agreement on what causes pyloric stenosis.
- Increasing choice of the medical way of treating PS with anti-acids rather than surgery.
- One day (keep dreaming?) the consignment of pyloric stenosis as a problem for newborns and their families.
- Reducing the post-operative and long-term after-effects after pyloromyotomy.
- Progress in the avoidance and treatment of post-surgical adhesions.
- The growing recognition of medical trauma in childhood, infancy, and adulthood as a cause of post-traumatic stress.
- Increased awareness world-wide about the sentient-ness (awareness of extreme life events) of preemies, neonates and infants.

The ancient Greek Plato summarised this essay well and a long time before it was written and read:
The greatest mistake in the treatment of diseases is that there are physicians for the body and physicians for the soul, although the two cannot be separated.

Contributing Author:
Frederick L Vanderbom, B.A. (Hons) University of Tasmania, Hobart, Tas.;
Th.Grad. (Reformed Theological College, Geelong, Vic.);
fred.vanderbom@gmail.com

Fred Vanderbom was born in the Netherlands in 1945 and his family migrated to Australia in 1951. He obtained degrees in Arts at the University of Tasmania and theology at the Reformed Theological College in Geelong, both in Australia. He worked in Christian churches in 3 Australian States from 1971 – 2010 and during this time also served as a hospital and aged care chaplain, in mission administration, as his denomination's historian, and as a school board chair. Since retiring from paid work he and his wife have been able to spend more time with their far-flung children and other family, and also to devote more time to several of his special interests: walking, swimming, gardening, photography, blogging, and shipping history and modelling.

Abstract

The large majority of infant pyloromyotomies are quickly successful and have few or no significant continuing effects. The lay author argues on the basis of his own and others' experience that for a small number of subjects there are ongoing consequences and pleads for more consideration and research to establish the numbers involved and a suitable response.

Endnotes

[1] Vanderbom, F.L. (2010-2014), Surviving Infant Surgery (WordPress Blog),
http://survivinginfantsurgery.wordpress.com/

[2] Krogh, Camilla, Biggar, Robert J., Fischer, Thea K., Lindholm, Morten, Wohlfahrt, Jan, and Melbye, Mads (2012), Bottle-feeding and the Risk of Pyloric Stenosis, *Pediatrics*, originally published online September 3, 2012. DOI: 10.1542/peds.2011-2785,
http://pediatrics.aappublications.org/content/early/2012/08/28/peds.2011-2785.full.pdf

[3] McAteer J.P., Ledbetter, D.J., and Goldin A.B. (2013), Role of bottle feeding in the etiology of hypertrophic pyloric stenosis, *JAMA Pediatriacs*. 167(12):1143-9. doi: 10.1001/jamapediatrics.2013.2857.
http://www.ncbi.nlm.nih.gov/pubmed/24146084

[4] My post, (2011), A survivor by accident,
http://survivinginfantsurgery.wordpress.com/2011/01/11/a-survivor-by-an-accident/

[Type text]

[5] Anand, K.J.S. and HICKEY, P.R. (1987), Pain and its Effects in the Human Neonate and Fetus, *The New England Journal of Medicine*, Volume 317, Number 21, pages 1321-1329, 19 November 1987.
http://www.cirp.org/library/pain/anand//

[6] My post (2012), Pyloromyotomy has made progress,
http://survivinginfantsurgery.wordpress.com/2012/10/11/pyloromyotomy-has-made-progress/

[7] Paul, Annie Murphy (2008), The First Ache, *The New York Times Magazine*, Feb 10,2008.
http://www.nytimes.com/2008/02/10/magazine/10Fetal-t.html?_r=1&ex=12

[8] F. Schier, F. (2008), Universität Mainz, Germany. Kinderchirurgie, Vorlesung Pylorushypertrophie.
http://www.unimedizin-mainz.de/Kinderchir/presentations/pylorushypertrophie.pdf

[9] http://onlinelifelines.blogspot.com.au/2006/11/this-is-tamara.html"
Svea Boyda-Vikander, Life Lines, 2 Nov 2006

The Cause

My Story—Ian Rogers.

Personal History-Gastrin and Acid.

I graduated MB. Ch.B from Glasgow in 1967. After 3 years surgical training in Glasgow and in Westminster Hospital London I found myself back in Glasgow in 1970 on the slippery pole of a training in General Surgery at Glasgow Royal Infirmary.

In those days and no doubt even today, publications were a solid passport to success in a surgical career. Glasgow academics excelled in gastro-intestinal physiology, no doubt fuelled by the epidemic of morbidity and mortality of the consequences of duodenal ulcer, a condition in those days which was common and dangerous.

Hyperacidity was well understood to be the cause and aberrations of gastric physiology, either constitutional or acquired, were regarded as the moving force. The acid secreting part of the stomach was from the lining cells of the proximal part of the stomach-the parietal cells of the body and fundus.

Gastric acid secretion was known to be caused by both the activity of the vagus nerves (neural or anticipatory phase) and a chemical agent or hormone known as gastrin (the gastric phase).

Prof. Gregory had been able to extract gastrin from the mucosa (lining) of the antrum of the stomach. When this extract was injected intra-venously it caused an outpouring of gastric juice rich in acid. (1)

He called this chemical gastrin and, as it clearly travelled in the blood stream to cause effects at a distant place, it was indeed a hormone.

Subsequent investigations revealed that gastrin was present in the antral mucosa and was released most effectively by the distension of the antrum especially when the gastric contents were relatively alkaline and contained peptides (amino acids). (2)

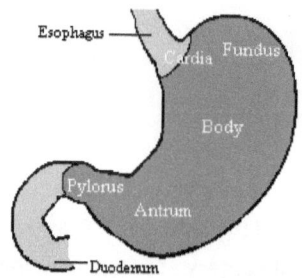

DIAGRAM 1.

Since both antral distension and alkalinity were both caused by food distending the antrum and neutralizing acid (the buffering effect), gastrin was secreted in response to food. The gastrin-induced acid was then available to start the gastric phase of digestion and to sterilize any bacteria introduced by food.

It was also known that there was a negative feedback between antral acidity and gastrin secretion-hence with high acidity, the gastrins were low and vice versa. After a meal, gastrin rises due to a temporary drop in antral acidity with associated antral distension. (3)

Thus in normal adult physiology acidity levels were not allowed to become too excessive- the upper limit and the lower limit was under gastrin control. It all made good physiological sense.

Histamine in a body weight (B.W.) dose of 0.01mgm/kgm subcutaneously was known to stimulate the secretion of gastric acid. However the results were not consistent.

In a practice-changing paper in 1953 Prof. Andrew Kay from Sheffield investigated the relationship between acid-response and histamine dose.

He clearly showed that maximal acid secretion required 4 B.W. doses of histamine i.e. 0.04 mgm/kgm. Histamine Test. Increasing the dose produced no greater response. In addition the dose response curve was s-shaped which indicated that the parietal cell secreted acid in an all or none way. Such findings allowed an interpretation of what was called the Parietal Cell Mass- the maximal ability to secrete acid. This extra large dose of histamine became known as the Augmented Histamine Test.(4) This Augmented Histamine Test revealed that adult males had a greater PCM than adult females-they secreted more acid(4)

Duodenal ulcer (D.U.) patients were by these means also shown to have a Parietal Cell Mass greater than normal. Their fasting gastrins were low to normal. (5)

D.U. patients also secreted more gastrin after a meal and there were relatively more G cells (gastrin producing cells) in the antral mucosa. This was especially true when the acid-induced duodenal ulcer had scarred sufficiently to produce a functional gastric-outlet obstruction-pyloric stenosis. (6)

In DU patients the male sex-ratio was 5:1. This sex-ratio was thought to be due to the known greater acid secretion in adult males.

The other main drive for acid secretion came from the activity of the vagus nerves. These nerves produced acid secretion from the brain whenever there was hunger or when food was anticipated.

The most usual cause of hyperacidity (and duodenal ulcer) was thought to be vagal- over activity . Over anxious male individuals were especially at risk.

Typically in cases of D.U., the basal acid output and maximal acid output was high and the fasting gastrins were not unexpectedly, low to low normal.

In those days before knowledge of H. Pylori or potent anti-acid treatment the reduction of acid was in the hands of the surgeon. If repeating the Augmented Histamine Test (A.H.T.) after a medical vagotomy (atropine and hexamethonium) revealed a big reduction in A.H.T., surgical vagotomy was indicated.

If there was only a small reduction then the antrum-the source of gastrin- was removed during a gastrectomy often combined with a vagotomy.

A small but potent pentapeptide of gastrin called pentagastrin is now routinely used parenterally in a body weight dose, to assess the maximum acid secreting ability of the stomach and hence the P.C.M.

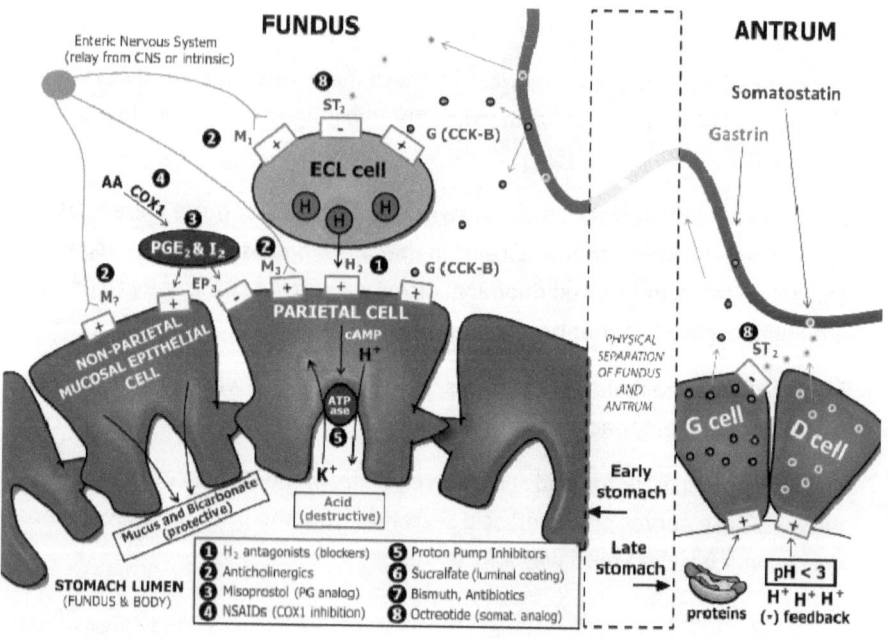

DIAGRAM 2.

This diagram outlines the way in which gastrin, released by amino acids/distension and alkalinity, travels by the blood from the antral mucosa to stimulate the parietal cell directly or indirectly through the ECL cell. Somatostatin travelling the same way and secreted from the D cells in response to an acid environment, inhibits this process as well as directly reducing secretion from the Gastrin cell through receptor ST2.

The vagus nerve stimulates the adjacent enterochromaffin like (ECL) cells to release Histamine which stimulates the parietal cell. The vagus nerve and its networks (enteric nervous system) can also stimulate the parietal cell directly or the mucous producing cells by using different receptors. A similar mucous effect occurs when Arachnodoic acid (AA) is converted into prostaglandins (PGE2 and I2) by the cyclooxygenase enzyme(COX 1). The secretion of mucous reduces the effect of acid and pepsin. NSAID drugs and aspirin inhibit the COX enzyme and hence can produce a gastritis. Classically the vagal phase or cephalic phase is responsible for 30% of acid secretion and the gastric or antral phase (gastrin secretion) 50%. Histamine and gastrin work synergistically.

Atropine will not block the release of gastrin from the antrum but it does block the vagal release of histamine from the ECL cell and, when given with hexamethonium produces a similar reduction as with vagotomy.(7).(8) By blocking the M1 receptors it stops the vagal neurotransmitter acetyl choline from releasing histamine from the ECL cell.

Also the histamine 2 receptors were now able to be blocked by H2 receptor blockers, such as cimetidine or ranitidine, with a considerably greater effect in reducing acid secretion.

Most importantly the final common pathway for acid secretion from the parietal cell is the proton pump mechanism whereby Potassium ions (K+) in the lumen are exchanged for Hydrogen ions (H+) from within the cell. Hence proton pump inhibitors such as Lansoprazole or omeprazole in adequate dosage completely abolish acid secretion.

On rare occasions the acid secretion would be high and the fasting gastrins would also be raised. There were 2 main causes.

1. Patients after a difficult gastrectomy in which part of the antrum containing the gastrin G-cell secreting part had been retained. Normally this would be removed. The retained antrum was then subjected to an alkaline bilious environment- a model for hypergastrinaemia and acid

ulceration of the anastomosis between stomach and jejeunum—stomal ulcer.

Gastrins and acidity were both high. The negative feed-back rule had been broken (9) and there was no gastrin control of acid secretion. (10) See Diagram 3

2. Patients with very rare tumours of gastrin producing cells elsewhere- frequently in the pancreas- called gastrinomas. These tumours presented with signs and symptoms caused by extreme hyperacidity such as repeated duodenal ulcer perforations. In this instance gastrins were very high indeed as was acidity. In addition because there was maximal uncontrolled gastrin secretion when fasting, there was no post-prandial gastrin rise.

Hence such findings in the absence of a gastrectomy and retained antrum, were diagnostic. Such a tumour became known as the Zollinger-Ellison (ZE) syndrome after the two researchers who first discovered the condition(11).

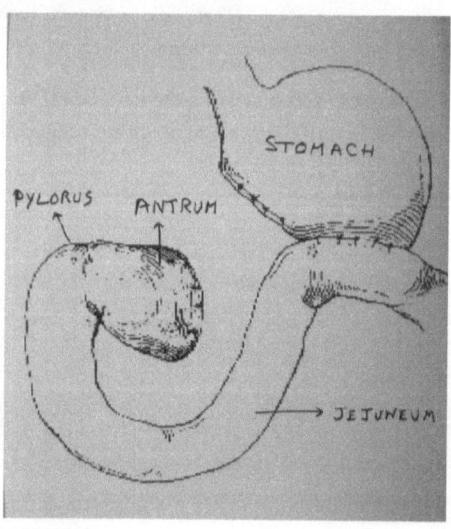

DIAGRAM 3.

However, the classical duodenal ulcer patient was likely to have the following features.

1. Male- sex ratio 5:1
2. High acidity.
3. A good appetite- they were hungry for food despite the ulcer.
4. Other affected members of the family.

Gastric outlet obstruction was also possible from fibrosis due to the ulcer. Even at this stage a medical cure could be achieved by timely Proton Pump inhibition.(12) The development of metabolic alkalosis through prolonged vomiting of acid was routinely also successfully treated by Proton Pump inhibitors or H2 receptor blockers.

All of these classical clinical features as we shall see, are uncannily similar to the classical features of Pyloric stenosis of infancy even including what John Thomson in his comprehensive account of 1921 described as the voracious appetite of the pyloric baby-- soon after vomiting the babies were eager for more feeds(13).

The huge contribution of Helicobacter pylori at this time to the causation of D.U. was not known. H. Pylori affects more than 80% of D.U. patients.

When the bacterium H. Pylori infects the lining of the stomach , it surrounds itself with an alkaline environment by secreting ammonia derived from urea in the tissue fluid. Hence it is protected from acid destruction. The local alkaline environment around the bacterium stimulates gastrin secretion from the antrum- and hence the general acid secretion in the lumen of the stomach is increases commensurate with the Parietal cell Mass.

Yet the huge preponderance of males with D.U.strongly suggests that H.Pylori is simply unmasking the known greater Parietal Cell Mass in adult males and thus producing acid induced duodenal ulceration. It has become known now that the frequency of H. Pylori infection in males and females is almost the same.

Although infrequent in youth the incidence approaches 70% in adults over 60 years.(14)

This then was the state of our knowledge in 1972 when I returned to Glasgow Royal Infirmary as Rotating Registrar in Surgery and started a 3 month attachment to the Paediatric Surgical Unit at Stobhill Hospital under the supervision of the late John Grant FRCS, Consultant Paediatric Surgeon.

The Cause of Infantile Hypertrophic Pyloric Stenosis.

The Clinical Clues.

It is an adage oft repeated-and certainly true. Listen to the patient-he is telling you the diagnosis. So must it be with the cause of infantile hypertrophic pyloric stenosis .(IHPS)

The infant is certainly very generous with his clues.

The presentation at 3 weeks of age-

the 5/1 male predominance-

the natural cure with time if temporary medical treatment is survived—(13)

the strong familial tendency-(15)

the complete disappearance of the tumor after simply dividing the hypertrophied sphincter – (13)

the high acid secretion which is not explained by acid accumulating behind a closed pylorus(16)(17) the high (unstimulated)basal acid output(BAO) and acid disease in long term survivors-(18)(19)

the voracious appetite.(13)

the persistence of the tumor in the thriving baby after gastroenterostomy (20)(21)-

the repeated observation of primogeniture (first –born baby more often affected)---(22)

the presence of superficial duodenal ulcers in some babies.(22a)(22b)

All these observations should combine to make the process easy. (see Figure 1)

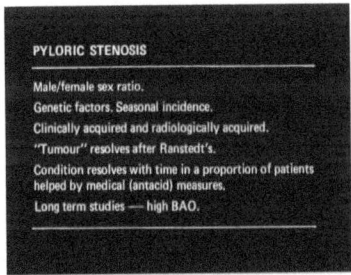

FIGURE 1

Many medical and surgical detectives have no doubt pondered the problem and yet the cause remains completely unknown 120 years after IHPS was first reported.

The Historical Setting.

In an important paper from 1921, Dr. John Thomson of the Royal Hospital for Sick Children, Edinburgh reviewed 100 cases of IHPS during the previous 25 years 1894-1919 . 58 had ended fatally. In patients surgically treated in Hospitals, rather than in Private Practice, the mortality was a staggering 75% (21 deaths) compared to 18.2%(2deaths) in private practice. The same findings obtained also with medical treatment. Ramstedt's operation(pyloro-myotomy) resulted in only one death out of 5 patients. The cases which recovered were all operated on by Sir Harold Stiles- the first exponent of pyloro-myotomy 6 months in fact before the eponymous Conrad Ramstedt.(see Image 2)

John Thomson made the following observations

1) The tumour was in fact a true muscular hypertrophy of the pylorus.
2) The disease is self-limited. He echoed the words of Robert Hutchison-that the pyloric lumen will eventually open up spontaneously and the child recover completely provided he does not die in the process.
3) Feeds must be restricted to 2 oz. or less and there should be warm water wash-outs once or twice a day. When babies had been treated with unsuitable feeding it was of the greatest importance to stop all feeding for 24 hours and use sub-cutaneous saline infusions,
4) He recognized categories of IHPS- an *acute* form with sudden and violent symptoms: an *ordinary* form and(most importantly) the *very mild case*. He described these cases as not at all uncommon. They probably resolve simply by dietary restriction alone and may never come to medical attention.

In a perceptive analysis of cause he debates the two main theories. I quote-

"Is the abnormal action of the pylorus a secondary phenomenon, due to the muscular coat being primarily affected by a simple congenital redundancy of growth as Hirschsprung and others have suggested? Or is the functional abnormality to be regarded as the primary element in the process- the muscle

being hypertrophied merely because- from an early period it has been worried into overgrowth by constantly recurring overaction—such as would result from even a slight degree of habitual incoordination?"

John Thomson favoured the second possibility-that of sphincter work hypertrophy. He cited the work of the great anatomist John Hunter, who in the 18th. Century had pointed out that a tendency to hypertrophy as a result of repeated forcible contractions is" a property of all muscles" and is greater in involuntary than in voluntary muscles. It is also extremely probable that tissue growth of this sort is specially active in early infancy(13).

In the beginning, therefore, in this the most common cause of neonatal upper GI obstruction, pylorospasm and indeed work hypertrophy from repeated contraction, was the favored explanation. (2) This theory silently lapsed presumably for want of corroborative data.

It is perhaps unsurprising to find that a condition very similar to IHPS has been reported in mammals- especially dogs (23).

My Journey.

Neonatal gastrin and acidity.

37 years ago as a young surgical trainee, I came across the 1947 paper by Miller in which he documented the seemingly unrelated phenomenon of neonatal hyperacidity.

Miller measured free and total acidity from 50 healthy mature breast fed infants 7 hours after their last feed, from day 1 to day 10. Samples after day 10 were collected from infants who were available at the time and the collection involved far fewer infants and was essentially random.

He reported that the immediate post-partum gastric neutrality due to swallowed amniotic fluid, became quickly hyperacid after a few hours and remained so for several days. Miller proposed the trans-placental passage of a chemical from mother(or placenta) to baby at the time of birth, which would cause secretion of foetal gastric acid as an explanation. It would be 10 years before gastrin, the hormone which causes gastric acid secretion was discovered by Gregory. Miller was indeed looking into the future(24).

Indeed he further found that from day 10 onwards it slowly increased. Miller supposed that this slow increase was due to the infant taking over control of acid secretion. Futhermore, the difference between maximum and minimum acidity after the 10th. day diminished with time.

The concept of a relative insensitivity between emerging gastrin and antral pH which is later explained below, is supported by his observations.

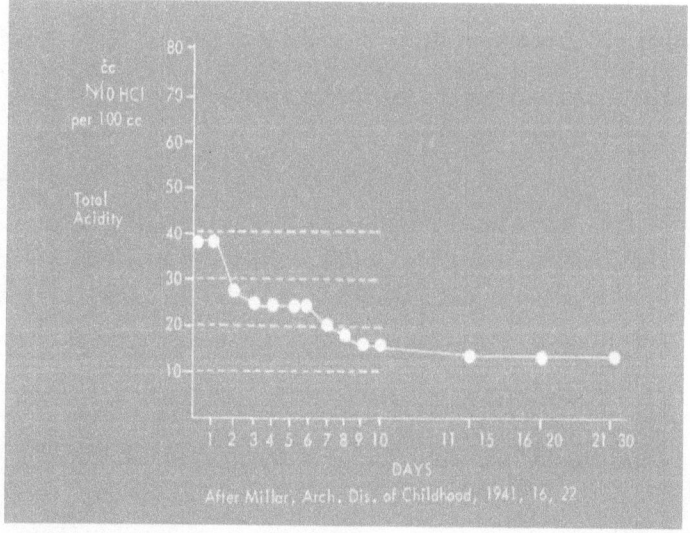

FIGURE 2   GASTRIC ACIDITY FROM BIRTH (after Miller 1941)

The above graph only measures total acidity with an endpoint to phenolphthalein(pH.10) <>10.) **When free acid (pH <> 4) is considered it correlates directly with the birth weight . Free acid fell to zero in most cases** *after the second day of life and the maximum acidity in fasting juice was probably reached within 24 hours of birth.*

An early increase in acidity has been confirmed by others.(25)(26)

Our attempts to prove gastrin transfer at birth, while non-confirmatory as far as maternal transfer was concerned, clearly showed for the first time that fasting gastrin levels rise from birth to very high levels at 4 days of life(27). Indeed the fasting levels at day 4 were higher than fasting adult levels.

Gastric juice at the moment of birth is usually alkaline because of swallowed amniotic fluid and subsequent studies have revealed that gastric acidity is present by Day 4. Hence the rising gastrin at a time of rising acidity strongly suggests that gastrin is the cause of the acidity and consequently, potent(28).

Neonatal hypergastrinaemia from Day 4 onwards to about 2 months of age when it levels off, have been reported and confirmed by others. (29), (30) (31)(32)

The cord level of gastrin was generally higher than the peripheral fasting maternal venous level. However later mammalian studies have revealed that the human placenta tissue concentrations are very high at the time of birth.

Indeed gastrin is known to cross from mother to baby in dogs and to cause acid secretion(33). Hence maternal transfer from human mother to baby via the placenta, is quite possible and was not excluded by this study. Fig.3. Fig.4.

Maternal gastrin rises progressively during pregnancy and peaks at labour. The maternal placenta is very rich in gastrin and the placenta is a likely source of elevated gastrin levels at birth with neonatal gastric acidity and growth of the stomach as an additional benefit(34). Within 30 minutes of delivery the maternal plasma gastrin is known to fall(35).

Sheep experiments in which metabolic clearance rates and production rates of gastrin were measured, have established that foetal production of gastrin continues to rise from 2 weeks before birth onwards.(36)

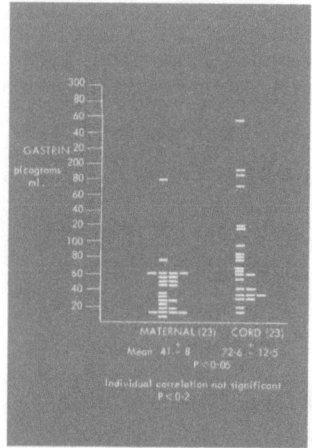

FIGURE 3 Maternal fasting venous gastrin levels and cord gastrin at birth.

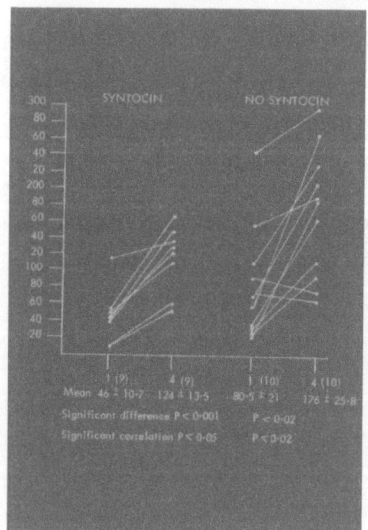

FIGURE 4. Cord gastrin levels at birth(Day 1) and fasting venous levels Day 4.

Some labours were promoted and augmented by syntocinon injection and when separately analysed there was an individual correlation between Day and Day 4 only in the syntocinon group. One explanation is that gastrin transfer occurs in the spontaneously born child and syntocinon inhibits this transfer. In this syntocinon group the cord gastrin was significantly reduced.($p<0.001$) Fig.4.

Pyloric sphincter contraction.

The entry of acid into the duodenum is known to be a potent stimulus to pyloric sphincter contraction in human adults and in dogs. (37)(38).
When intravenous gastrin is given to adults, the first consequence is pyloric delay (presumably from pyloric contraction) (39).
In adults with hyperacid disease, the early symptom of post-prandial bloating (pyloric delay), is quickly relieved when acid secretion is abolished by timely antacid therapy. Indeed, selected cases of pyloric stenosis in adults have been shown on occasions to be successfully managed by antacid therapy alone. (12).

The physiology of gastric emptying in the adult.

When food enters the adult stomach, the stomach behaves functionally as if it had a proximal and a distal half.

The fundus and body acts as a reservoir progressively relaxing to accommodate the volume of food with little increase in pressure. There are 3 phases to this which are effected by non-adrenergic/noncholinergic (NANC) vagal pathways.

1. Receptive relaxation controlled by anticipatory reflexes related to swallowing and chewing.
2. Adaptive relaxation- caused by local gastro-gastric reflexes/chemoreceptors/mechano-receptors.
3. Feedback relaxation-caused by receptors from the digestive part of the small intestine.

After a meal in the *digestive phase*, *tonic* small amplitude contractions will empty the food into the antrum where *cyclical* phasic peristaltic waves (the antral pump) propel the food bolus(chyme) towards the pylorus in **Phase 1** of the fed pattern activity..

In **Phase 2** the liquid chyme is partly expelled through the pylorus since the middle antrum contractions induce a relaxation of the pyloric sphincter. More solid chyme escapes backwards through the still open contracting antral ring proximally to the body of the stomach- the phase of emptying and mixing. The pylorus contracts with contraction of the terminal antrum in this Phase-hence there is a churning action , enabled by pyloric contraction, to make sure that only fluid chyme exits the pylorus.

In **Phase 3** the contracting antrum continues to act against a closed and contracted pylorus and propels the chyme backwards towards the body in a grinding fashion- all of which is designed to make the food particles smaller before propelling them through the pylorus like a sieve. This fed- pattern activity is characterized by maximum frequency low amplitude contractions of the pyloric sphincter.

The pyloric sphincter contracts frequently in response to hydrochloric acid (or oleic acid)entry with a frequency determined either by the duodenal or the antral frequency of contractions- presumably to prevent duodeno-gastric reflux. The known release of cholecystokinin by acid entering the duodenum is thought to be a hormonal cause of pyloric contraction.

The *interdigestive phase of gastric motility* on the other hand, functionally cleans out the stomach and coordinates in sequence with intestinal peristalsis. Pyloric sphincter relaxation is coordinated with antral peristalsis.(see the GI Motility tutorial)

Hence pyloric sphincter contraction is a phenomenon particularly associated with feeding.

Motilin is a recently discovered peptide hormone located in the duodenal mucosa. It is released when the duodenum is empty and induces the gastric part of the Migrating Motor Complex(MMC) **inter-digestive phase**. **Phase 3** of the MMC features the hunger contractions – or so called rumbling of the stomach 4 hours after a meal which empties the stomach before the next meal. Emptying of course requires a pylorus still capable of being opened.

The frequency of gastric contractions is determined by a network of cells called **Interstitial cells of Cahal (ICC)** which cause the local smooth muscle cells to contract by the opening up of Calcium channels using cholinergic excitatory neural pathways. The pylorus is an electric isolator such that the frequency of duodenal peristaltic contractions occurs at a higher and different rate.

Whatever the complex fine detail, it is perfectly clear that repeated feeding produces repeated pyloric sphincter contraction which is further increased in frequency and force in hyperacid states. The ***fed pattern*** gastric activity requires the pylorus to contract when antral peristalsis presents incompletely digested feeds to it. It would be difficult for an inexperienced mother to resist the temptation to feed her vomiting baby who is again clamoring for a re-feed.

Readers interested in knowing more about pyloric sphincter physiology are directed towards the papers by H.J.Ehrlein and Michael Schemann on gastro-intestinal motility(40).

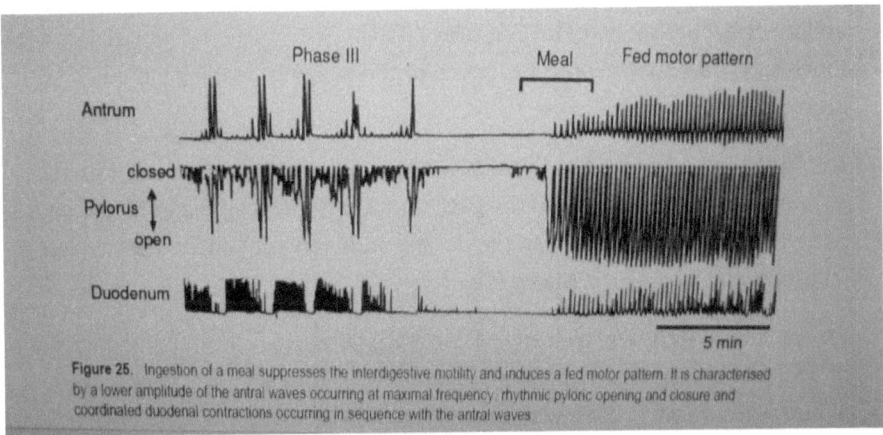

Figure 25. Ingestion of a meal suppresses the interdigestive motility and induces a fed motor pattern. It is characterised by a lower amplitude of the antral waves occurring at maximal frequency; rhythmic pyloric opening and closure and coordinated duodenal contractions occurring in sequence with the antral waves

FIGURE 5. (Reproduced from the Tutorial on Gastro-intestinal Motility H.J.Ehrlein and M. Schemann by permission from M.Schemann).

Pressure tracings contrasting the difference between pyloric contractions in Phase 111 of the interdigestive motility pattern and the fed pattern. The fed pattern is clearly associated with more frequent sphincter contractions.(From Gastro-intestinal Motility Tutorial) (40)

Gastric function and the Hyperacidity Theory.

What would happen if adult physiology also applies to the proposed pathogenesis of pyloric stenosis of infancy?

Milk feeds accumulating behind a closed sphincter would produce temporary antral alkalinity with antral distension, both classical causes of gastrin secretion.(28)Thus the resulting gastrin-induced acidity would potentially lead to repeated sphincter contraction, work hypertrophy and , in due time an enlarged hypertrophied and pyloric sphincter-in short IHPS.

Whether this happens or not would depend on the potential acid secreting ability –the inherited Parietal Cell Mass.(PCM). Too much acid would mean too much sphincter contraction. Too much or too frequent feeding would accelerate the process.

Artificial mechanical narrowing of the pylorus in rats with a ligature, has been shown to stimulate growth of the gastric mucosa; increase the PCM and cause hypersecretion of acid through the double stimulation of an increased gastrin level and an increased PCM.(41)(42).

Hence pyloric stenosis by itself in infants will produce further active secretion of acid with an even greater encouragement to more acid-induced work hypertrophy. Gastrin itself was considered to be a possible culprit since it was also capable of inducing pyloric contraction either directly (43) or indirectly through the acid secreting effect. (See Diagram 4.)

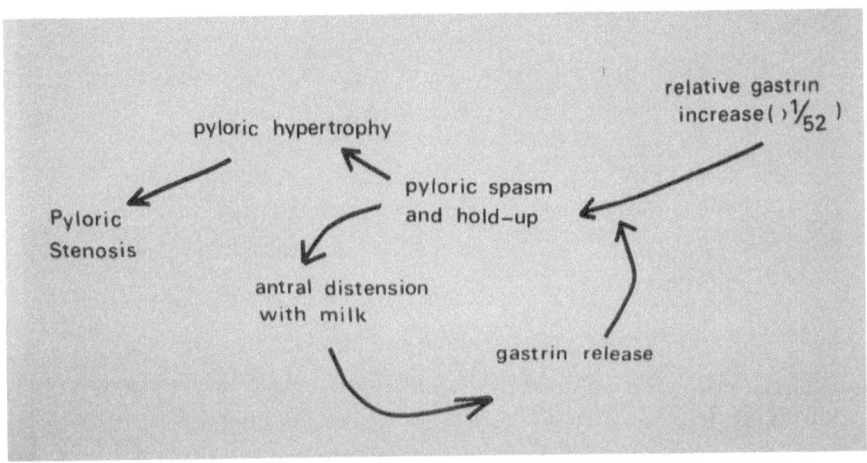

DIAGRAM.4. Early Theory of Causation. From Rogers et al.–Pyloric stenosis a gastrin hypothesis disproved?(44)

This early gastrin theory was investigated by measuring fasting gastrins in IHPS babies and matching controls. We established that fasting gastrin levels were statistically no different in the babies with IHPS (44) . Most other authors reported similar findings apart from Spitz who reported higher fasting gastrins after a shorter 4 hour period of fasting(45).

Curiously and intriguingly post-prandial gastrin levels after pyloro-myotomy are generally reported to be higher than normal(46).(47)

Subsequent larger studies from research laboratories have refuted the earlier findings of the gastrin effect on the circular sphincter. The consensus is that cholecystokinin and secretin contract the sphincter- presumably released by duodenal acid(48).

Gastrin or its synthetic pentapeptide pentagastrin contracts the circular antral muscles(49) and relaxes the pyloric sphincter in animals(50) and this relaxing effect has been confirmed by sphincter pressure measurements in human volunteers.(51).

Hence gastrin induced hyperacidity now remained the main and only suspect.

IHPS and Acid secretion.

In our study, all the parameters of acid secretion-volume; basal acid secretion (titration to pH 4) and total acidity(titration to pH 10)was greatly increased (17) compared to matched controls.

The increased hypersecretion of acid in IHPS has been confirmed using Histamine stimulated acid studies both before and, most importantly, 1 week after pyloromyotomy. (16)

Thus the increased acid secretion is real- and not due to a normal acid secretion accumulating behind a closed pylorus and being inadequately emptied by the initial aspiration. Others have acid hypersecretion in IHPS simply on the basis of much lowered pH levels after a 6 hour fast(18.)

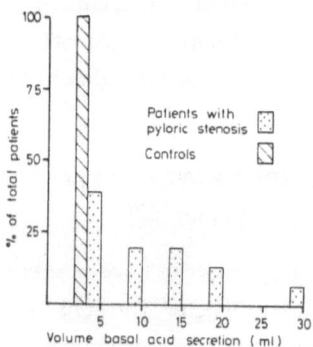

Fig. 2 *Basal acid secretion.*

FIGURE 5. Free Acidity. Only IHPS babies had measurable free acidity.

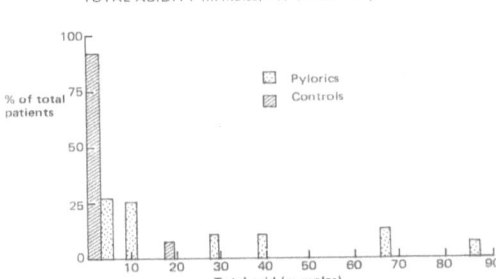

FIGURE 6 Total Acidity.

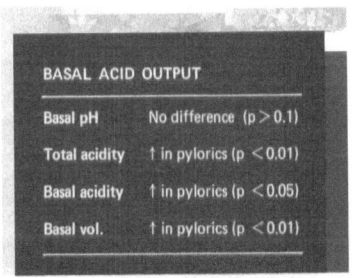

TABLE 1

Soon after this paper was published, I discovered the work of Prof. John Dodge. He had been able to produce pyloric stenosis in new-born puppy dogs by giving injections of pentagastrin (a synthetic substitute for gastrin) to their mothers before birth. 28% of puppies were affected and 16% of these were found at post mortem examination to have superficial pyloric ulceration. (52) Fig.7.

Even more puppies developed pyloric stenosis when the pentagastrin injections were given to them after birth.

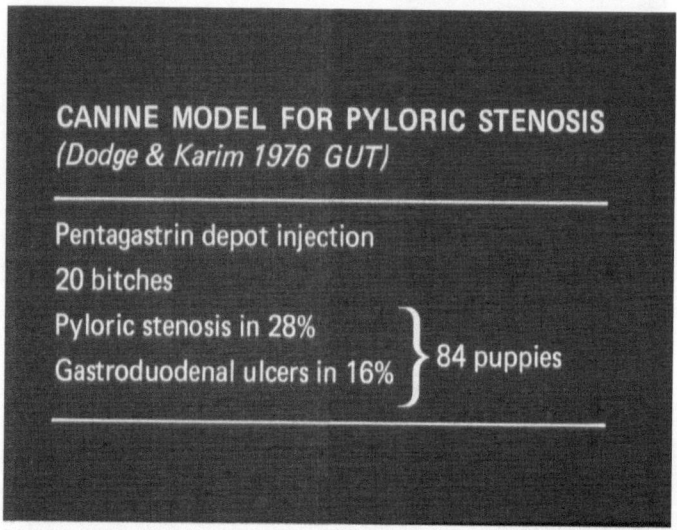

Figure 7.

An explicit interpretation was not given but pentagastrin-induced acid secretion in the puppy appears the most likely cause particularly since it is known that gastrin crosses the canine placenta and stimulates acid secretion. (33)(Figure 7).

Sphincter Work Hypertrophy as the Cause.

The place of the sphincter, is clearly integral to the cause.
Divide the sphincter- the tumour disappears. Bypass with a gastroenterostomy and it remains.
Hence an intact contracting sphincter is essential and incriminates work hypertrophy as the culprit.
These observations should similarly exclude any proposal that muscle growth from genetically determined aberrations of growth factors have a part to play.

Any muscle which enlarges due to repeated contraction does so by means of attracting growth factors. The various growth factors reported in the hypertrophied sphincter muscle by Puri and others in several papers, signify only that the muscle is enlarging from repeated contraction- nothing more. It is not support for a primary contribution from abnormal or aberrant growth factors(53).

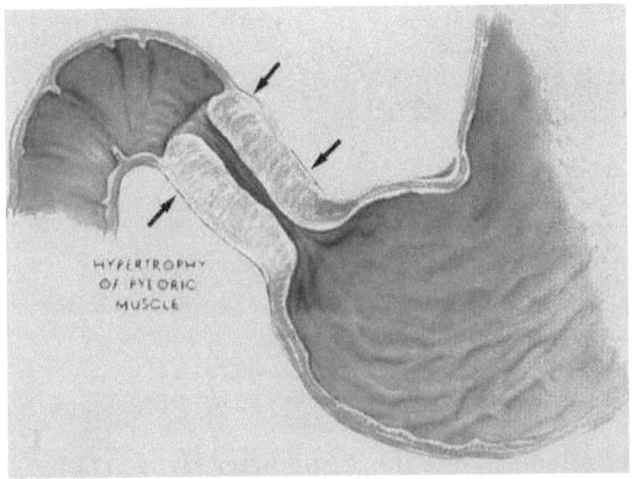

DIAGRAM 7. IHPS-an artist's impression.

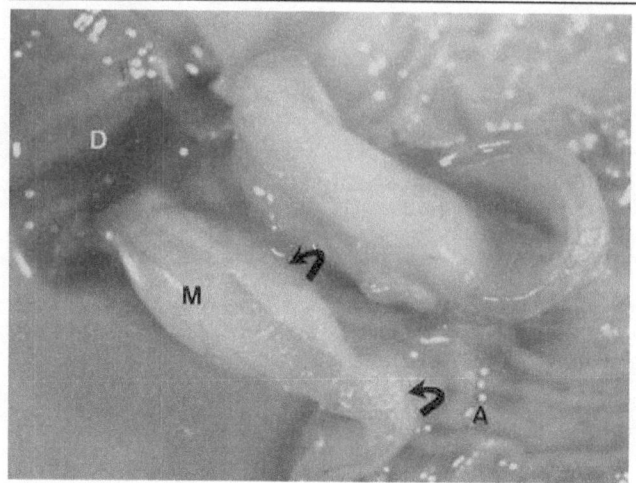

IMAGE 1. Real life picture of Pyloric Hypertrophy and Stenosis. A =antrum, M=sphincter muscle, D =duodenum

The Anatomy and Pathology of Pyloric Sphincter Hypertrophy and Stenosis.

Histological study of the pyloric tumour has confirmed muscle hypertrophy as the cause of the tumour(54).
Other reported histochemical abnormalities of many sorts have also been reported. All the quantitative chemical reports rely on a comparison with autopsy controls at various times after death, Hence no true comparison is actually possible.
Pathological abnormalities described are similarly going to be much influenced by the huge distorting muscle hypertrophy requiring for example larger neural elements for proper sphincter function(55).
Electron microscopic observations of the tumour tissue has revealed no abnormalities(56).

Sphincter work-hypertrophy is also supported by the erythromycin phenomenon.

A 7-fold increase in the incidence of IHPS has been reported among newborn infants who received erythromycin in antibiotic doses for post-exposure pertussis prophylaxis. (57).

Erythromycin, a macrolide antibiotic with motilin like activity, specifically increases antral motility (58) and contraction of the pyloric bulb (59) (60) by binding to motilin receptors.

These receptors not only exist in cholinergic nerves but also are thought to exist directly on smooth muscle. The strongest antral contractions induced by large doses of erythromycin are not blocked by atropine and direct muscle stimulation is likely. (61)

Indeed the authors of the pertussis report (54) specifically speculate that that the marked gastric motility leads to (work) hypertrophy of the pylorus.

The Motilin Story.

The gastro-intestinal hormone motilin is responsible for the mass emptying movements of the stomach in the inter-digestive phase when the stomach should be empty(Migrating Motor Complex MMC). It is classically secreted from the duodenal mucosa when the duodenum is empty or alkalinized (62)(63)(64).

The voltage-tension curves for the antral-pyloric region coupled with the narrow pyloric diameter at this age mean that the interdigestive phase 2 contractions may encounter a closed pylorus under the influence of erythromycin.

More recent reports have shown that duodenal pH does not influence endogenous motilin release if the pH is between 2 and 8.5 (65), a range well within the pH range in IHPS. (18)

Nutrients in the duodenal cap strongly suppress the typical pulsed interdigestive motilin release. (66) and clearly this means that the motilin release in babies with IHPS will not be restricted. Others have produced evidence that acid in the duodenum also liberates motilin(67). This matter is still unclear.

However the empty duodenum in IHPS whatever the pH may provide a means whereby motilin maintains the stimulus of pyloric sphincter contraction through the M.M.C. of the interdigestive phase.

It is of further interest to record that motilin plasma levels rise steeply after birth in normal infants reaching levels greater than those in fasting adults by day 24 and that the motilin and the post-natal increase of gastrin, require that the infant be fed (30).
The one report of motilin levels in IHPS record low levels. (68) and further corroborative analyses are clearly required.
An analysis of the motilin gene (MLN) has compared normal controls with babies with IHPS and no mutations or differences have been detected. (69).

Clinical Aspects.

The standard confirmatory test for a baby of the right age, who has copious non-bilious vomiting is *the standard test meal.*

The clinician sits to the right of the baby who is often lying comfortably on mothers lap after a feed. Gentle epigastric palpation reveals the characteristic pyloric tumour in about 80% of babies with IHPS. Associated post-feed gastric distension and left to right peristalsis may be viewed as further confirmation (see images from Dr. Vanderbom).

Studies in **adults** with an active duodenal ulcer (and presumed hyperacidity) have shown that interdigestive Phase 3 expulsive contractions which empty the stomach ,require acid-blocking drugs to alkalinize the antral contents. (68)(69). These interdigestive contractions are characterized by antral contractions occurring when the pylorus is relaxed. Hence the potential for gastric emptying in IHPS simply as a result of ranitidine (H2 receptor blocker) therapy, appears well-founded.

Fed-pattern contractions on the other hand, will also increasingly meet with a closed pylorus as the condition develops- a scene well known to those who have felt the contracting tumor in the classical test feed.
Hence the baby who inherits a high PCM will because of developmental acid drive in the first few weeks of life, develop uncontrolled hyperacidity which would translate into regular sphincter contractions.
This will be especially true if the first time mother re-feeds the obviously hungry baby through a natural anxiety.

A recent decline in the incidence of IHPS that parallels the decline of sudden infant
death (SIDS) has been observed in Sweden, which coincides with the implementation of the —back to sleep campaign in an attempt to reduce the frequency of SIDS (70).
Gastric emptying is likely to be increased by the supine position compared to the prone position since duodenal emptying in the prone position requires feeds to move against gravity.
Hence the back to sleep phenomenon at least has a physiological basis .
An improved emptying would allow acid secretions to pass normally through the open pylorus during the critical developmental first few weeks and antral distension would be avoided.

Personal career considerations as a General Surgeon then intervened and my own contribution came to an end in the late 1970s.

Clinical Questions resolved.

At around 1990 I revisited the problem anew. The following persistent questions all prompted by the same clinical features, still remained unanswered.

1. What makes some babies develop IHPS when normal babies do not?

2. Why do male babies predominate?

3. Why self-cure with the passage of time?

4. Why is it more frequent in the first born?

5. Why does pyloromyotomy, and not gastro-enterostomy, cause the tumor to disappear? (1)

6. Why does it present at around 3-4 weeks of age?

Question 1.

What makes some babies develop IHPS.?

The only certain observed abnormality up till this time was hyperacidity. What if an inherited primary **hyperacidity**, that is acidity at the top of the normal distribution curve, were the primary cause? Indeed, when viewed from the perspective of a proposed **primary inherited hyperacidity**, many observations are explained..

For example one need no longer ponder on the relatively normal fasting gastrin levels. Indeed if the gastrin negative feed-back is functioning at this age(and this is by no means certain) the hyperacid PS baby ought to have lower gastrins. Their normality is not a problem and indeed their normality may even point to a relative gastrin excess- since it should be lower.

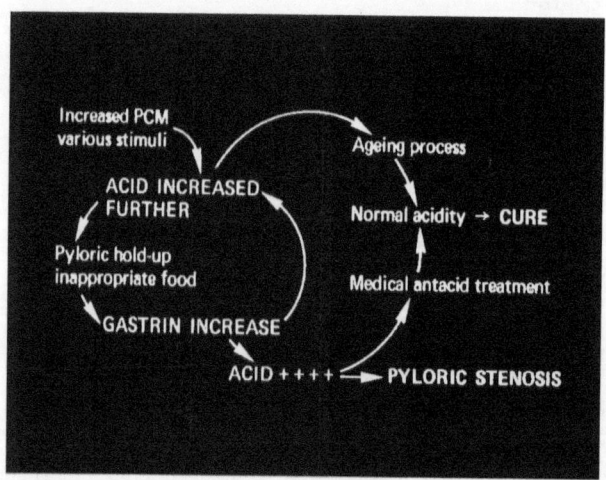

Diagram 9. Pathogenesis of IHPS based on an Increased Parietal Cell Mass.(PCM) with inappropriate continued feeding as a further stimulus.

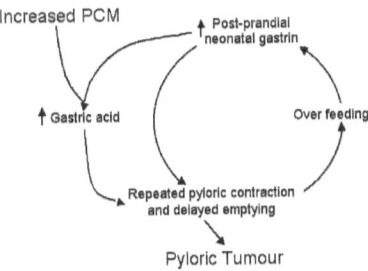

Diagram 10.

Pathogenesis of IHPS based on Primary Hyperacidity and post-prandial gastrin increase.

Studies of fasting gastrin and post-prandial gastrin in babies with IHPS have revealed no difference compared to normal infants, either before or after operation.(71) One caveat is that it would be difficult to distend the artificially enlarged(but emptied antrum) before surgery with a feed of normal volume. Hence gastrin release may be less than in the usual repeated feeding scenario.

Any baby in the pyloric age group who persistently vomits and who is alkalotic, is invariably found to have IHPS. (72).
This obvious implication of active hyperacidity in IHPS confirms our earlier laboratory investigations.

It is indeed part of this theory that there will be babies who slip in and out of gastric outlet obstruction and who may never come to the doctor's attention. The process of work hypertrophy will be in balance with both the gradual fall in hyperacidity and the gradual widening of the pyloric lumen with time,
This group would conform to Thomson's *very mild cases* which in his experience was not at all uncommon(13).

Supporting evidence for hyperacidity.

1. Oesophageal atresia.

The repeated finding of a tenfold increase in IHPS in babies with esophageal atresia (73) supports the hyperacidity theory. The early possibly gastrin-induced acidity will not be alkalinized by swallowed liquor in the majority of these cases. Thus the foetus is theoretically exposed to greater acidity before and after labour and the possibility of IHPS gets a head start. Feeding for obvious reasons is also delayed so mounting gastric acidity remains unbuffered in the early post-natal days.

2. Long term acid studies after IHPS.

Adults who have had IHPS have been shown repeatedly to suffer from the adult consequences of hyperacidity such as duodenal ulcer with high volume acid secretion and are subjected more often to peptic ulcer surgery. (74)

Babies destined to develop IHPS would inherit an acid secreting ability towards the top of the normal range. The simple reason for this would be the inheritance of a greater parietal cell mass than normal. Both duodenal ulcer patients and babies with IHPS, share a preponderance of the O blood group which, particularly when a non-secretor status, is associated with hyperacidity. (75)(76).

Consequently the strong familial multifactorial inheritance would be explained.(77)

Babies with a normal acid secreting ability would have insufficient acid, despite the developmental hypergastrinaemia in the first weeks, to trigger the process.

Question 2.

Why male babies?

The male predominance is also explained. The male/female sex ratio of 4-5/1 parallels the sex-incidence of duodenal ulcer in adult males- a condition known to depend on hyperacidity and to depend on a large PCM.

Mary Ames in 1959 investigated the gastric acidity in the first 10 days of life in 58 pre-term babies weight 1000-2,200gm. The endpoint of Topfers reagent and phenolphthalein was used to determine free and total acidity respectively.

> Initial specimen was obtained within 12 hours of birth and subsequently 6 hours after the last feed. 43 babies were able to be assessed at day 10.

> The average free and total acidity was determined for each day . The formula feed was half-skimmed milk and corn syrup. The greatest acidity in the whole group occurred on the 4th day of life.

> In the first 5 days of life the total acidity from boys averaged 51.2 units compared to 39.1 in girls.

> The second 5 days figures were 61.1 in boys compared to 35.2 in girls.

Pre-term male babies thus have been clearly shown to have more total acid than matched females (78). This report published in 1959 remains unchallenged.

Ethical considerations may prevent further naso-gastric studies in normally-fed term babies.

Question 3.

Why self cure with time.?

Important analyses of the relationship between neonatal gastrin and acid secretion in normal babies provide a credible explanation of the phenomenon of self-cure.
Sequential studies of fasting and post-prandial gastrin were performed up to 4 months of life in normally developing infants.

Fasting gastrins remain significantly high at 2 months of age compared to maternal levels and there is no post-prandial gastrin response.

> At 3 and 4 months the pattern appears to revert to an adult pattern with statistically significant post-prandial elevations.
> After 2 months of age the fasting gastrins are a little lower and a post-prandial gastrin response can be detected. (29).
>
> The authors explain these findings on the basis of a **relative insensitivity** of the gastrin-acid relationship in the first few weeks of life. By this they mean it has not matured sufficiently to respond inversely to antral acidity. Similar findings of high fasting gastrins within the first few days of life with no post-prandial increase has also been reported from the same laboratory(79).

Hence between birth and 3 weeks the *normal* baby exhibits some of the biochemical findings of a temporary Zollinger-Ellison syndrome(ZE).(11)
Fasting gastrin is being maximally secreted commensurate with developmental imperatives and cannot be further increased by food.

It also cannot be reduced when the expected rise in gastric acidity occurs. Hence gastric acid secretion is temporarily increased.
For the baby with a normal parietal cell mass(PCM) this is of little consequence- but for a baby with a PCM at the top end of normal, dangerous hyperacidity with IHPS as a consequence is a real possibility.(see Diag. 11 and 12)

This phenomenon is the presumed explanation for peak acidity in *normal* development at between 10-17 days reported and graphically outlined by Agunod (80) in a pivotal paper.

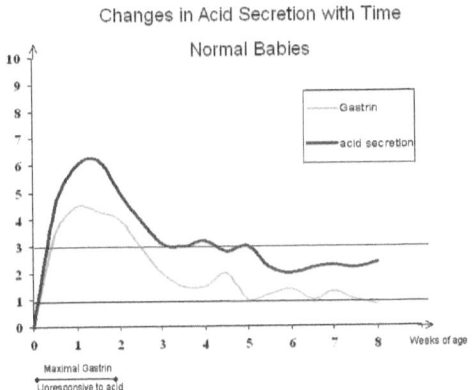

Diagram 11. Probable Relationship between acid and gastrin in normal babies.

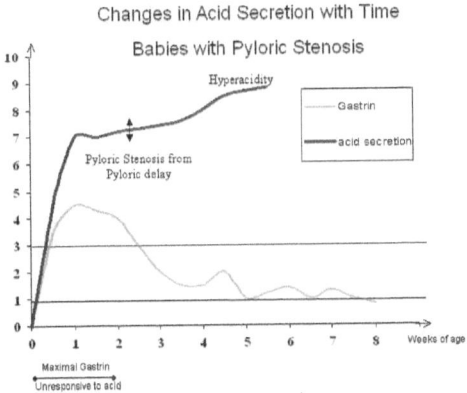

Diagram 12. Proposed Relationship between acid and gastrin in babies destined to develop IHPS

Babies who inherit a large P.C.M. will trigger the process of pyloric stenosis when hyperacidity is temporarily increased from birth to 2-3 weeks of age.

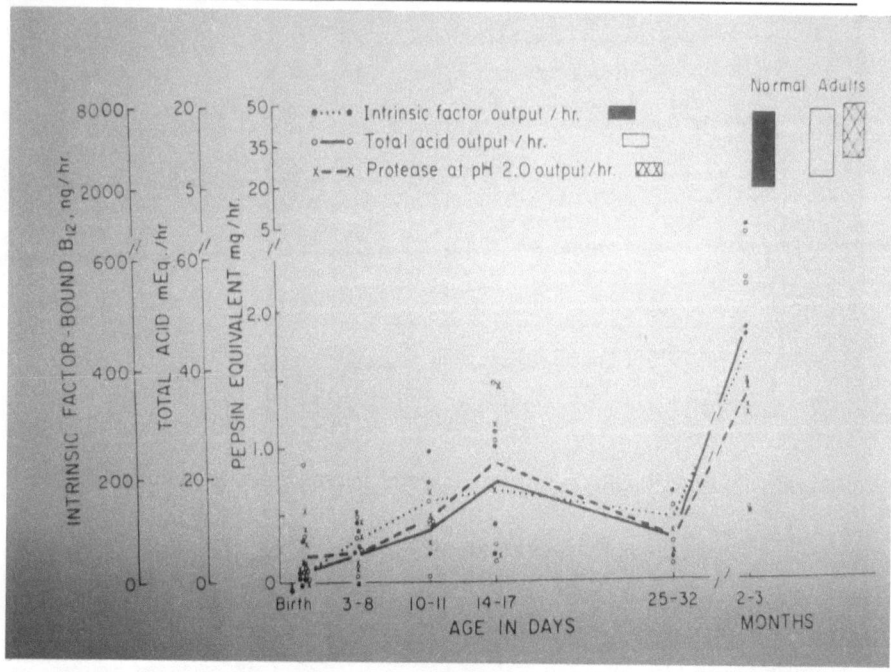

Figure 8. After Agunod. The rise in all 3 gastric parameters , gastric pepsin, intrinsic factor and acid secretion peaks at between 14-17 days.(80)

Hyman and others studied 34 healthy preterm infants once a week during hospitalization. They also reported that both basal and peak acid secretion increased to a plateau around 4 weeks.

Basal acid output, pentagastrin-stimulated acid output, fasting serum gastrin, and fasting serum pancreatic polypeptide were measured during each study.

Basal acid output at 1 week of age was 12 µmol/kg/hr, increasing over the first 4 weeks to 30 µmol/kg/hr.

Administration of pentagastrin 6 µg/kg subcutaneously increased acid output in all age groups. Pentagastrin-stimulated acid output at 1 week was 21 µmol/kg/hr, increasing over the first 4 weeks to 44 µmol/kg/hr. Acid secretion did not change significantly over the next 4 to 6 weeks.

Fasting serum gastrin concentration was stable over the first 6 weeks of life, but doubled during the end of the second month. These studies confirm that the majority of healthy preterm infants secrete acid in quantity sufficient to maintain the gastric pH ≤4, providing an acid barrier to most gastro-intestinal bacterial pathogens (81).

The studies perhaps more importantly confirm Agunod's observation that acid secretion peaks at around 3-4 weeks of age.

Hence the baby who inherits hyperacidity is especially liable to trigger IHPS within the first few weeks of life . These infants have become in essence, a mini -ZE syndrome with a hyperacidity not able to be reduced by a functioning adequate negative gastrin feed-back. (11)

Untreated the condition will usually lead to a fatal outcome.

Pyloromyotomy will provide a quick long-lasting cure by stopping work-hypertrophy and allowing acidity to be naturally reduced by peristalsis and by a matured controlling negative feed-back with time.

The medical treatment hallowed by tradition was based on the proposal that spasm of the sphincter was the problem and that atropine, an anticholinergic spasmolytic, would help. The vagus nerve-which is classically contracts the smooth muscle of the gut and whose final mediator is acetyl choline, was thought to be involved in pyloric spasm. Hence the anticholinergic atropine was used.

The present understanding of the place of acetyl choline in gastric motility and acid secretion provides a rationale for the success of atropine in the medical therapy.

Hence temporary medical treatment using atropine and gastric wash-outs, not only reduces acidity by reducing the vagal drive but also physically removes gastric acid by suction and by reducing antral distension. The baby is thus kept alive until the developmental time sensitive drive to hyperacidity has passed.

Other supportive measures such as relief of dehydration and control of fluid balance and acid-base balance are also clearly required.

With time the gastrin/acid negative feed-back matures and the pyloric canal widens relative to the feeds.

Hence with the developmental acid drive now over, the acid secretion comes under gastrin control. The natural widening of the pyloric canal with time ensures that a long lasting cure is achieved with temporary medical treatment.

Question 4.

Why more frequent in the first-born?

The first born child is fed by a first-time mother. Vomiting babies, especially IHPS babies classically are hungry and vigorous babies and are classically able to take more feeds soon after vomiting.. The inexperienced mother, no doubt is a more anxious mother and is more likely to continue to feed the baby who vomits.

The stomach will be seldom allowed to be empty. Hence the process of feed-promoted and acid-induced work hypertrophy of the pylorus would continue. A more experienced mother is likely to give the stomach a rest.

The work of Jacoby is of particular interest in this matter. Although a pediatrician, he treated IHPS both surgically and medically. A similar mortality of 1% in 100 surgical and 100 medically treated babies was reported. Great stress was put on the need for *relative under nutrition* as part of the well controlled body weight dosage of atropine therapy in the medically treated group. Regular gastric washouts to empty the stomach was also part of the medical treatment(82).

The very low reported incidence of IHPS in underdeveloped countries may also reflect infrequent overfeeding but many other factors may be involved.(83)

Question 5.

Why does the tumour disappear after pyloromyotomy and not after gastro-enterostomy?

Pyloro-myotomy renders the sphincter incompetent and widens the lumen. Hence further contraction and work hypertrophy is impossible and the tumor quickly disappears.

Gastroenterostomy, the earliest surgical treatment, only bypasses the obstruction. The pathogenetic processes are only partially abolished.

Hence it is easy to understand why 52 years after gastroenterostomy the tumor has been shown to be still present (84)(13).

Question 6.

Why do symptoms appear at around 3-4 weeks of age?

On first principles there are 2 potential reasons why acid induced hypertrophy appears so typically at 3-4 weeks.

1. The acid stimulus occurs at birth and takes 3 weeks to produce sufficient work hypertrophy to qualify for a clinical diagnosis of IHPS. This remains a possibility. There is no need for immaturity of the negative feed-back mechanism in this mechanism.

If this were true more primary acid related problems should emerge at an early stage- in the first few years of life- and they do not.

2. The emerging neonatal hypergastrinaemia rising so quickly after birth- does by itself suggest that the negative feedback is not operating fully at this age given the known rise in acidity from birth to 3 weeks of age.

There is evidence which supports an insensitivity of the normal negative feed-back at this age. (29)

It makes good physiological and evolutionary sense that the feed-back starts to become normal after 3 weeks. Developmental hyperacidity is a good safeguard for the normal child- but it is dangerous for the baby with already too much acid.

Whatever the genetic inheritance is that produces an enhanced P.C.M, it is allowed to persist in the community, since the mortal challenge from too much acid is confined to a critical potentially survivable few weeks.

An inadequately performing negative feed-back by producing an early peak of acid secretion allows babies to defend themselves against early bacterial assault on the gut. The positive evolutionary aspects of this may well outweigh the negative evolutionary consequence of IHPS . Hence the genes which produce a large PCM survive.

Other contemporary lines of enquiry.

The Genetic Story.

Recent genetic analyses set up to explore the possibility of a monogenic association have simply confirmed the heterogeneous genetic inheritance is the norm.(85)(86) The concordance rate in monozygotic twins while greater than that in dizygotes, is still only between 0.25 and 0.44.(87)

The basic consensus is that IHPS remains a condition which is multigenic and multifactorial- the likely acceptable pathway for the inheritance of constitutional hyperacidity(77).

A detailed analysis of birth weight and gestational ages of babies who develop IHPS has revealed that they tend to have greater birth weight which is not explained by a longer gestational age. 148 IHPS babies' records were analysed.

The author was suggesting that these babies were more muscular and, indeed, there is anecdotal evidence that they more commonly become athletes (88).

Growth Factors and Chemical Agents.

The reported abnormalities within the pyloric sphincter muscle of various growth factors as well as deficiencies of other chemical agents such as nitric oxide synthetase, although theoretically attractive, do not stand up to critical analysis.(89). (Nitric oxide which is created in the tissues by nitric oxide synthetase starts a chemical process which relaxes endothelial smooth muscle –the muscle in the wall of small blood vessels).

Firstly, for obvious reasons, adequate control specimens are never going to be ethically possible. Age matched control specimens of pyloric sphincter muscle invariably consist of post-mortem tissue at various, sometimes unstated, times after death. Thus no proper comparison is possible.

Secondly, the reported accumulation of growth factors in the tumor tissue is no more than one would expect from a work-hypertrophied sphincter. When a repeatedly contracting muscle or a muscle subjected to an increasing load, becomes hypertrophic, it does so by attracting growth factors. (90)(91). There is no evidence to support genetically controlled inappropriate accumulation of growth factors as a primary process.

Thirdly- as with all the genetic studies there is no attempt to solve the dynamic mystery created by the many clinical clues these babies provide.

The Infection Theories.

The search for a necessary time-sensitive temporary environmental precipitant in pathogenesis has led to speculation about self-limiting infection

Throat swab analysis of the common nasopharyngeal viruses has shown no greater frequency in pyloric babies compared to normal matched controls(92).

Helicobacter pylori (H Pylori), the most important gastric pathogen and known stimulant of gastric acid secretion (93) has also been investigated.

H. Pylori is known to be present in some babies from 6 months in age. In a 5 year follow-up study of mother and child random amplified polymorphic D.N.A fingerprinting has revealed that mother to baby transmission does occur (94)

In another study prompted by an index case suspicion of H. Pylori organisms on histology, 16 consecutive babies with IHPS underwent gastric biopsy pre-operatively. All the urease tests for H. Pylori were negative, 4 cases had chronic gastritis, 6 had a mild gastritis and 5 were normal. No H. Pylori were discovered on histology (95).

At the age of pyloric presentation immunological tests for H. Pylori are unreliable since maternal transmitted immunity may last up to 6 months.

A further study using stool culture for H Pylori in 39 consecutive babies with IHPS failed to discover a single case. Control babies were also negative. (96)

Curiously the major consequence of H. Pylori infestation in adults- namely hyperacidity - is not mentioned as a possible link between infection and the development of IHPS in any of the cited papers.

In the absence of a known cause the gastritis recorded on biopsy presumably would simply be a consequence of prolonged gastric stasis.

There is consequently no evidence at present to support an infectious cause.

Conclusion

So there it is. My journey is almost complete. Constitutional hyperacidity coupled with developmental hyperacidity begets pyloric contractions which begets work hypertrophy which begets IHPS. IHPS begets further hyperacidity and so on.

Maternal anxiety in the novice mother means that the hungry but vomiting baby is frequently fed with more pyloric contractions and more work hypertrophy- and a bigger tumour.

We are almost back where we began so many years ago when Thompson in 1921 first proposed pylorospasm and work hypertrophy as the cause and Freund in 1903 had declared that a hydrochloric acid content in excess of normal was a causative factor in spasticity of the pylorus. (21- cited on page 485)(97)

There is, indeed ,nothing new under the sun.(21- page 485).

The Future.

This theory is perfectly testable. IHPS babies lose lots of acid when they vomit. The alkalosis may cause serious hypoventilation with anesthetic problems and a failure to breathe post-operatively. An adult similarly affected would be appropriately treated with the currently super-effective acid-blocking drugs with an immediate reduction in fluid, acid and potassium loss. Recently success has been reported with a quick reduction in tumour size by the use of intra-venous atropine in addition to standard medical treatment (98).

Indeed Banieghbal has already shown that intra-venous cimetidine (Histamine receptor 2-blocker) rapidly corrects the metabolic alkalosis of IHPS. Safe same-day surgery may then be undertaken without the usual 4 day delay to allow standard resuscitation fluids to reduce the alkalosis.(99)

Even more interesting is the yet unpublished data which shows that when intra-venous cimetidine is given to babies with established IHPS but with muscle thickness of 3 mm. or less, 16 out of 17 babies are completely cured by this means alone.(100)

The more powerful acid blockade by intravenous ranitidine(another H2 blocker) has also been shown to work in this age group(101) and should be even more effective in the early case or when surgery is not easily accessible.

Such a pre-operative strategy with babies with IHPS is long overdue. It should not come as a surprise if we find that such temporary treatment promotes a lasting cure.

In the adult version of IHPS, namely duodenal ulcer , ranitidine , perhaps by the induction of a motilin response, has been shown to significantly increase the rate of gastric emptying for solids and liquids.(102).

The even more powerful acid-blocking proton pump inhibitors omeprazole and lansoprazole have also been shown to work in the neonatal period and should be the ideal medical solution.

References.

1. Gregory R.A.,Tracy H.J. The constitution and properties of two gastrins extracted from hog antral mucosa. GUT, 19645, 103-117.

2.McGuigan JE, Trudeau WI. Studies with antibodies to gastrin. J.Physiol(Lond). Radioimmunoassay in human serum and physiological studies. Gastroenterology 1970; 58: 139-50.

3. Mahklouf GM, McManus JPA, Card WI. Action of pentapeptide ICI50 123 on gastric secretion in man. Gastroenterology 1966; 51:455-65.

4. Kay A.W. Effect of large doses of histamine on gastric secretion of HCl. B.M.J. 1953, July 11, 77-80.

5. Baron J.H. Studies of basal and peak acid output with an augmented histamine test. GUT ,1963, **4,**136-144.

6. Tani M., Shimazu H. Meat-stimulated gastrin release and acid secretion in patients with pyloric stenosis. Gastroenterology 1977,**73,** 207-210.

7. Gillespie I.E., Kay A.W. Effect of medical and surgical vagotomy on the augmented histamine test in man. B.M.J. 1963 June 3, 1557-1560.

8. Konturek S.J., Oleksy J., Wysocki A. Effect of atropine on gastric acid response to graded doses of pentagastrin and histamine in DU patients before and after vagotomy. Amer. J. Digest. Dis. 1968, 13(9), 792-800.

9. Wheeler M.H. Progress report. Inhibition of gastric secretion by the pyloric antrum. Gut. 1974, **15,** 420-432.

10. Burhenne H.J. The retained gastric antrum. Preoperative roentgenologic diagnosis of an iatrogenic syndrome. Amer. J.Rontgenology. 1967, 101, 459-67.

11. Zollinger RM, Ellison EH (1955). "Primary peptic ulcerations of the jejunum associated with islet cell tumors of the pancreas". *Ann. Surg.* **142** (4): 709–23.

12. Talbot D.. Treatment of adult pyloric stenosis: a pharmacological alternative? BJCP 1993; 47: 220-221

13. Thomson J. Observations on congenital hypertrophy of the pylorus. Edin.Med. J.1921; 26: 1-20.

14. Murray L.J., MacCrumm E.E., Evans A.E., Bamford K.B. Epidemiology of H.Pylori infection among 4742 randomly selected subjects from Northern Ireland. Int. J. Epidemol. 1997, 26(4), 880-887.

15.Mitchell L.E.Risch N. The genetics of IHPS. A reanalysis. Am.J.Dis. Child 1993:147:1203-11.

16. .Heine W., Grager B., Litzenberger M., Drescher U. Results of Lambling gastric juice analysis (histamine stimulation) in infants with spastic hypertrophic pyloric stenosis. Padiatr. Padol. 1986; 21: 119-25

17. Rogers I.M., Drainer I.K., Dougal A.J et al . Serum cholecystokinin, basal acid secretion and infantile hypertrophic pyloric stenosis .Arch. Dis. Childhood. 1979; 54: 773-75

18, Shinohara K., Shimizu T., Igarashi J., Yamashiro Y. Miyano T. Correlation of prostaglandin E2 production and gastric acid secretion in Infants with Hypertrophic Pyloric Stenosis. J.Ped. Surg.1998, 33, 1483-1485.

19. Wanscher B., Jensen H.E. Late follow-up studies after operation for congenital pyloric stenosis. Scand. J. Gastroenterol 1971, 6, 597-9

20. Dickinson S.J.,Brant E.E.Congenital pyloric stenosis. Roentgen findings 52 years after gastroenterostomy Surgery 1967, 62, 1092-4

21. Mack H. C. A history of hypertrophic pyloric stenosis and its treatment. Bull. Hist. Med. 1942, X11, 3 465-615.

22. Webb AR, Lari J.,Dodge J. Infantile hypertrophic pyloric stenosis in South Glamorgan 1970-79. Arch. Dis. Child. 1983,58,586-90.

22a. Harrison L.P.(1931) Arch. Dis. Child.,6,245.

22b. Holt L.E.(1913) Am.Jour. Dis. Ch. 6, 245.

23. Bellenger CR,Maddison J.E.,McPherson G.E. Ilkiw JE Chronic hypertrophic pyloric gastropathy in 14 Aus. Vet.J. 1990:67,317-20.dogs.

24. Miller, R. A. Observations on the gastric acidity during the first month of life. Archives of Disease in Childhood, (1941), 16, 22.

25. Davidson D.C., Rogers I.M., Ardill J., Buchanan K.D. Neonatal gastric hyperacidity. Further analysis of the oxytocin effect . 1976 Arch. Dis. Child.

26. Avery G.B., Randolph J.G., Weaver T. Gastric acidity on the first day of life. Pediatrics 1966, 37, 1005-7.

27. Rogers I.M., Davidson D.C., Lawrence J et al Neonatal secretion of gastrin and glucagon. Arch. Dis. Child. 1974; 49: 796-801.

28. Waldum H.I., Fossmark R., Bakke I., Martinsen C., Qvigstad G. Hypergastrinaemia in animals and man: causes and consequences. Scand.J.Gastroenterol. 2004; 39:505-509.

29. Moazam F., Kirby W.J., Rodgers B.M., McGuigan J.E. Physiology of serum gastrin production in neonates and infants. Ann Surg. 1984, April, 389-392.

30. Lucas A., Adrian T.E., Christofides N., Bloom S.R., Aynsley-Green A. Plasma motilin, gastrin and enteroglucagon and feeding in the human new born. Arch. Dis. Child. 1980, 55, 673-677.

31. Euler A., Byrne W. Cousins L.M.,Ament M.E., Leake R.D., Walshe J.H. Increased serum gastrin concentrations and gastric acid hyposecretion in the immediate newborn period.

32. Sann L., Chayyvialle A.P., Bremond A., Lambert R. Serum gastrin in early childhood. Arch. Dis. Child. 1975, 50, 782-785.

33. Bruckner W.L., Snow H, Fonkalsrud E.W. Gastric secretion in the canine foetus following maternal stimulation: Experimental studies on placental transfer of insulin, histamine and gastrin. Surgery 1970; 67: 360-363.

34. Attia R., Ebeid A.M., Fischer J.E./ Goudsouzian N.G. Maternal foetal and placental gastrin concentrations. Anaesthesia 1982, 37, 18-21.

35. Attia R.R., Ebeid A.M., Murray P., Fischer J.E. The placenta as a possible source of gut peptide hormones. Surg. Forum 1976, 27, 432-34

36. Shielkes A., Chick., Hardy K.J. Foetal and maternal production and metabolism of gastrin in sheep. J. Endocrinology 1982.,2, 183-189.

37. Cook A.R. Duodenal acidification: Role of the first part of the duodenum in gastric emptying and secretion in dogs. Gastroenterology . 1974; 67: 85-92

38. Fisher R.S, Lipshutz W, Cohen S. The hormonal regulation of the pyloric sphincter function. J. Clin. Invest.1973; 52:1289-1296.

39. Hunt J.N.,Ramsbottom N. Effect of gastrin 11 on gastric emptying and secretion during a test meal. Br. Med. J 1967; 4: 386-390.

40. Ehrlein H., Shemann Gastro-intestinal motility. http://humanbiology:wzw.tum.de/fileadmin/Bildertutorials.pdf

41. Crean G.P., Hogg D.F., Rumsey R.D.E Hyperplasia of the gastric mucosa produced by duodenal obstruction. Gastroenterology, 1969; 56:193-199

42. Omura N., Kashiwagi H., Aoki T. Changes in gastric hormones associated with gastric outlet obstruction. An experimental study in rats. Scand. J.Gastro. 1993; 28(1):59-62.

43. Rogers IM., MacGillion F.,Drainer I.K.D. Congenital hypertrophic pyloric stenosis . A gastrin hypothesis pursued. J. Pediatr. Surg. 1976,11,173-5.

44. Rogers I.M., Drainer I.K., Moore M.R. et al Plasma gastrin in congenital hypertrophic pyloric stenosis. A hypothesis disproved? Arch. Dis Child. 1975, 50(6), 467-471

45. Spitz L., Zail S.S.. Serum gastrin levels in congenital hypertrophic pyloric stenosis. Journal of Pediatric Surgery. 1976, **11**, 33-35.

46. Barrios V., Urrutia M., Hernandez M., Lama R., Garcia-Nova, Hernanz A, , Errila E. Serum gastrin level and gastric somatostatin content and binding in long-term pyloromyotomised children. Life Sciences, 1994, **4** ,317-325.

47. Bleicher M.Shandling B., Zingg W., Karl H., Track N.S. Increased serum immunoreactive gastrin levels in idiopathic hypertrophic pyloric stenosis. Gut, 1978,**19**,794-797.

48.Isenberg J.I., Csendes A. Effect of octapeptide of cholecystokinin on canine pyloric pressure. Amer. J. Physiol. 1972, 222,428.

49. Bennett A., Misiewicz J.J., Waller S.L. Analysis of the motor effects of gastrin and pentagastrin on the human alimentary tract in vitro. Gut. 1967, 8,470.

50. Isenberg J.I., Grossman M.I. Effect of gastrin and S/C 15396 on gastric motility in dogs, Gastroenterol.1969, 451.

51. Fischer R.S., LipshitzW.,, Cohen S..The hormonal regulation of pyloric sphincter function.. J. Clin. Invest. 1973., 52,1289.

52. Dodge J.A., Karim A.A. Induction of pyloric hypertrophy by pentagastrin.Gut. 1976; 17: 280-284.

53. Oshiru K., Puri P. Increased insulin-like growth factor and platelet –derived growth factor in the pyloric muscle in IHPS. J. Ped. Surg. 1998, 2, 378-381.

54. Oue T., Puri P. Smooth muscle hypertrophy versus hyperplasia in IHPS. Pediatr. Res. 1999, 45, 853-57.

55. Rogers I.M. New Insights on the pathogeneesis of pyloric stenosis of infancy. A review with emphasis on the hyperacidity theory. Open J. of Pediatrics. 2012, 2, 1-9.

56. Jona J.Z. Electron microscopic observations in IHPS. J. Pediatr. Surg. 1978,134,17-20.

57. SanFilippo A. Infantile hypertrophic pyloric stenosis related to the ingestion of erythromycin estolate: A report of five cases. J. Pediatr. Surg. 1976; 11: 177-180.

58. Honein M.A, Paulozzi L.J, Himelright I.M. et al. Infantile pyloric stenosis after pertussis prophylaxix with erythromycin: A case review and cohort study.Lancet 1999: 354: 2101-2106.

59. Di Lorenzo C, Flores A F, Tomomamas T et al. Effect of erythromycin on antroduodenal motility in children with chronic functional gastrointestinal symptoms. Dig. Dis. Sci. 1994; 39:1399—1404

60. Boiron M., Dorval E, Metman E.H, et al. Erthromycin elicits opposite effects on antro-bulbarand duodenal motility:analysis in diabetics by cineradiography. Arch. Physiol Biochem.1997;105:591-595

61. Coulie B, Tack J, Petters T, Janssens J Involvement of two different pathways to the motor effects of erythromycin on the gastric antrum in humans. Gut. 1998;43: 395-400.

62. Brown J.C., Johnson C.P, Magee D.F. Effect of duodenal alkalinisation on gastric motility. Gastroenterology 1966; 50: 333-339.

63. Kusano M, Sekiguchi T, Nishioki T. et al. Gastric acid inhibits antral phase3 (MMC) activity in duodenal ulcer patients. Dig. Dis.Sci. 1993; 38:824-831.

64. Itoh Z. Review. Motilin and clinical application. Peptides. 1997; 18:593-608.

65. Mori K, Seino Y, Yanaihara N et al. Role of the duodenum in motilin release.Regul. Pept. 1981; 1: 271-277.

66. Mitznegg P, Bloom S.R,Domschke W. et al. Release of motilin after duodenal acidification. Lancet 1976; 11: 888-889.

67. Segikuchi T, Kusano M, Nishioki T et al. gastroduodenal motor dysfunction and plasma motilin concentration in patients with duodenal ulcers. In Itoh Z. Ed.(60)Motilin. San Diego: Academic Press. 1990; 226-245.

68. Christofides N.D, Mallet E, Bloom S.R. Plasma motilin in IHPS. Biomed.Res. 1982; 3: 571-572

69. Svenningson A, Lagenstrad K, Omrani M.D, Nordenskjold K. Absence of motilin gene mutations in IHPS . J. Ped. Surg 2008; 43: 443-446.

70. Persson S, Ekbom A, Granath F, Nordenskjold A. Parallel incidence of sudden infant death syndrome and infantile hypertrophic pyloric stenosis. Pediatrics 2001;108. E70.

71. Moazam.F., Rodgers B.M.. Talbert J.L., McGuigan .Fasting and post-prandial serum gastrin levels in Infants with Congenital Hypertrophic Pyloric stenosis.

72. Maizels M. Alkalosis in the vomiting of infancy. Arch. Dis. Child. 1931; 1:293-302.

73. Vilarino A., Costa E. Ruiz S. Association of oesophageal atresia and hypertrophy of pyloric stenosis. Cir.Esp. 1977: 31; 239-241.

74. Wanscher B, Jensen H.E. Late follow-up studies after operation for congenitalpyloric stenosis. Scand. J. Gastroenterol. .1971; 6: 597-9.

75. Koster K.H., Sindrup E. Seele V. ABO blood groups and gastric acidity. The Lancet, 1955,July 9 , 52-56.

76. Dodge J.A. ABO blood groups and IHPS. BMJ 1967, 4, 781-2.

77. Carter C.O. The inheritance of congenital pyloric stenosis. Br. Med. Bull.1961; 17: 251-254

78. Ames Mary .Gastric acidity in the first 10 days of life of the prematurely bornbaby. . Amer. J.Dis. Child. 1959; 2: 1123-1126

79. Rodgers B.M., Dix P.M., Talbert J.L et al. Fasting and postprandial serum gastrin in normal human neonates. J.Ped. Surg 1978; 13, 13-16.

80. Agunod M. Correlative study of hydrochloric acid, pepsin and intrinsic factor secretion in newborns and infants Amer. J. Digest Dis. 1969 ; 14: 400-13.

81.Hyman P.E., Clarke D.D., Everett S.L. et al. Gastric secretory function in pre-term infants. Pediatrics, 1985,106,467-68

82. Jacoby N.M. Pyloric stenosis. Selective medical and surgical treatment.Lancet 1962; (Jan), 119-121

83. Joseph T. P, Nair R. R. Congenital hypertrophic pyloric stenosis. Ind. J. Surg.1974; 36: 221-223.

84. Dickinson S.J., Brant E.E Congenital pyloric stenosis. Roentgen findings 52 years after gastroenterostomy. Surgery. 1967; 62: 1092-94

85. Chung E, Curtis D, Chen G et al. Genetic evidence for the neuronal nitric oxide synthetase gene (NOS1) as a susceptibility locus for infantile hypertrophic pyloric stenosis. Am.J. Hum genet. 1996; 58: 363-370.

86. Everett K.V, Chiosa B.A, Georgouls C et al. Genome-wide high density SNP-based linkage analysis of infantile hypertrophic pyloric stenosis identifies loci on chromosomes 11q14-q22 and Xq23. Am. J.Hum. Genet. 2008; 82:756-762.

87. Schechter R, Torfs C.P, Bateson T.F. The epidemiology of infantile hypertrophic pyloric stenosis. Paediatr.Perinat. Epidemol. 1997; 11: 407-427.

88. Czeizel A. Birthweight distribution in congenital pyloric stenosis. Arch. Dis. Child(1972, 47,978-980.

89.Subramaniam R.,Doig C.H.,Moore L. Nitric oxide synthetase is absent in only a subset of cases of pyloric stenosis. J.Pediatr. Surg2001, 36, 616-619.

90. Fath K. A, Alexander R.W, Delafontaine P. Abdominal coarctation increases ILGF im RNA levels in rat aorta. Circ. Res. 1993; 72: 271-277.

91. Hannson H. A, Jenmache E, Shottner A. IGFI expression in blood levels varies with vascular load. Acta. Physiol. Scand. 1987; 129: 165-169.

92. Mcheik J.N. Are viruses involved in IHPS? J. Med. Virol 1982; 12: 2087-2091.

93. Dahshan A, Donovan K.G, Halabi I.M. et al. Helicobacter Pylori and IHPS. Is there a possible relationship? J. Ped. Gastro. Nut. 2006;42:262-264.

94. Konno M, Fuji N, Yokota S et al. Mother and child transmission of H.Pylori J. Clin. Microbiol. 2005;43: 2246-2250.

95. Paulozzi L.J. Is helicobacter pylori a cause of IHPS? Med. Hypothesis 2000; 55:119-125.

96. Sherwood W, Choudhry M, Lakhoo K. Infantile hypertrophic pyloric stenosis: an infectious cause. Paediatr. Surg. Int. 2007; 1: 61-63.

97. Freund W.1903 Central.bl.f.d. Grenzgib.d.Med.u.Clin 11,309

98. Kawahara H., Imura K., Nishikawa M., Yagi M., Kubota.A. Intra-venous atropine treatment in infantile hypertrophic pyloric stenosis. Arch. Dis. Child.2002, 87,71-74.

99. Banieghbal B. Rapid correction of metabolic alkalosis in hypertrophic pyloric stenosis with intravenous cimetidine: preliminary results. Pedatr. Surg. Int. 2009, 25, 269-271.

100. Banieghbal. Personal communication. 2013.

101. Kelly E.J., Chatfield S.L., Brownlee K.G., Ngt P.C., Newell S.J., Dear P.R.F., Primrose J.N. The effect of intra-venous ranitidine on the intra-gastric pH of preterm infants receiving dexamethasone. Arch. Dis. Child. 1993, 69, 37-39.

102. Huscher C., Falchetti D., Besozzi F., Dessanti A. et al. Ranitidine and total gastric emptying of liquids and solids. Curr. Ther. Res. ,1984, 36, 916-920.

Acknowledgements.

The references here bear witness to the curiosity, discipline and imagination of many researchers who have, like me, have pondered on the cause of this most curious condition. My thanks are due to them.

My own journey and perceptions here outlined, have been encouraged and focused by their scientific observations.

My thanks are due to the late John Grant F.R.C.S., Consultant Paediatric Surgeon, Stobhill Hospital, Glasgow who first encouraged me to continue with these studies. Prof. Harold Ellis F.R.C.S., late Prof. Surgery, Westminster Hospital, London, has also been a source of general and specific encouragement.

Biographical Data.

Ian Rogers worked as a Consultant Surgeon at the Ingham Infirmary, South Shields and subsequently at South Tyneside Foundation Trust from 1978-2004.

He went to Allan Glen's School, Glasgow and qualified M.B., Ch.B. from Glasgow University in 1967.

Surgical Training was received at Glasgow Royal Infirmary and Westminster Hospital London.

He is the author of many papers on the cause of pyloric stenosis of infancy and other general surgical topics.

He was President of the North East Surgical Society of England in 2000 and was for many years a Guest Examiner in Surgery for the Royal College of Physicians and Surgeons, Glasgow.

After retirement he spent several years teaching Surgery at AIMST University in Malaysia as a Visiting Professor in Surgery.

Most of his retirement time is spent in music either as a choir member(Voices Together) or as singer in a musical trio, The Three Wise Men.

He is married with 4 children.

[Type text]

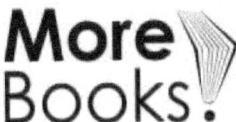
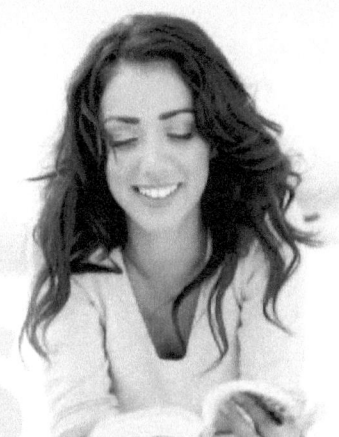

I want morebooks!

Buy your books fast and straightforward online - at one of world's fastest growing online book stores! Environmentally sound due to Print-on-Demand technologies.

Buy your books online at
www.morebooks.shop

Kaufen Sie Ihre Bücher schnell und unkompliziert online – auf einer der am schnellsten wachsenden Buchhandelsplattformen weltweit! Dank Print-On-Demand umwelt- und ressourcenschonend produziert.

Bücher schneller online kaufen
www.morebooks.shop

KS OmniScriptum Publishing
Brivibas gatve 197
LV-1039 Riga, Latvia
Telefax: +371 686 204 55

info@omniscriptum.com
www.omniscriptum.com

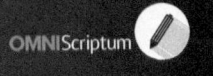

www.ingramcontent.com/pod-product-compliance
Lightning Source LLC
Chambersburg PA
CBHW031538210526
45464CB00003B/1068